Implementing Inquiry-Based Learning in Nursing

If you want to introduce Inquiry-Based Learning (IBL) into your curriculum but are not sure how to go about it, this book will set you on the right track. In *Implementing Inquiry-Based Learning in Nursing* the author shares the experience of leading a project to implement IBL as an integrated whole pre-registration curriculum and provides a blueprint for successful implementation.

The practicalities of implementing IBL can be a daunting prospect. Using a wealth of examples, relevant theories, models and research, this book takes the reader through the logistics of every stage of implementation. Part I provides the necessary theoretical and research perspectives. Part II describes in detail how to manage the project stage by stage, covering planning, implementation, evaluation and change management. Part III looks at the operational practicalities and describes eight subprojects: staff development; communication systems; the classroom compass; practice experience; documentation; electronic, library and media resources. Part IV reviews the post-implementation situation.

Whether you are new to or already familiar with Inquiry-Based Learning, or simply need some practical guidelines, this book will provide an indispensable source of reference.

Dankay Cleverly is the Inquiry-Based Learning Coordinator for the pre-registration nursing curriculum at Anglia Polytechnic University and Head of the Life and Social Sciences Division in the School of Health Care Practice. She has professional qualifications in both nursing and education and has been involved in curriculum development for more than a decade.

Implementing Inquiry-Based Learning in Nursing

Dankay Cleverly

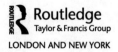

Routledge
Taylor & Francis Group

LONDON AND NEW YORK

First published 2003
by Routledge
11 New Fetter Lane, London EC4P 4EE

Simultaneously published in the USA and Canada
by Routledge
29 West 35th Street, New York, NY 10001

Routledge is an imprint of the Taylor & Francis Group

Typeset in Times by
Keystroke, Jacaranda Lodge, Wolverhampton
Printed and bound in Great Britain by
Biddles Ltd, Guildford and King's Lynn

British Library Cataloguing in Publication Data
A catalogue record for this book is available from the British Library

Library of Congress Cataloging in Publication Data
Cleverly, Dankay
    Implementing inquiry-based learning in nursing/Dankay Cleverly.
        p. cm.
    Includes bibliographical references and index.
    1. Nursing—Study and teaching. 2. Inquiry (Theory of knowledge)
    I. Title.
RT142 .C547 2003
610.73'071'1—dc21   2002031931

ISBN 0–415–27484–2 (Hbk)
    0–415–27485–0 (Pbk)

For my husband, Peter

Contents

PART IV
By the time tomorrow comes   129

Figures

About the author

Dankay Cleverly is the Inquiry-Based Learning Coordinator for the pre-registration nursing curriculum at Anglia Polytechnic University, and Head of the Life and Social Sciences Division in the School of Health Care Practice. She has professional qualifications in both nursing and education and has been involved in curriculum development for more than a decade.

Her work with inquiry-based learning extends to: a postgraduate module *Facilitating Inquiry-Based Learning* for which she is a facilitator; presenting papers at conferences and seminars locally, nationally and internationally; and external consultancy on implementing inquiry-based learning.

Preface

Aims of the book

We lived through a memorable experience at Anglia Polytechnic University: the successful implementation of inquiry-based learning (IBL) – during which we developed and field-tested a blueprint for implementing IBL. This account aims to provide a readable and practical guide for the intending student-centred learning project team and all academics, and other professionals, with an interest in the topic. The focus is on the operational aspects of implementing IBL in an integrated whole curriculum in a pre-registration nursing programme. However, the principles and much of the practical advice are directly applicable to all other student-centred inquiry- /problem-based learning programmes.

The book seeks to redress a perceived lack of literature on IBL. It puts forward a curricular philosophy supported by relevant theory and models. The original and adapted models in this book are freely available for review and critique. There is no intent to assert the rightness or otherwise of other curriculum implementations.

Curriculum development issues have not been discussed separately, since the focus of this book is on implementing IBL.

The generic term 'curriculum management group' is used throughout the book to represent several management groups with similar functions related to the project.

Key features of the book

The following are some of the features developed as a further elucidation of important aspects of the IBL implementation project:

- A conceptual framework and an eclectic model of metalearning for understanding IBL and its processes are provided in Chapter 3.
- Gantt charts are provided to show the scheduling of each of the eight subprojects in Chapter 4.
- Eight subprojects for implementing the operational aspects of the curriculum are reviewed in Chapter 5.
- A curriculum evolution model is presented in Chapter 15.

- A comprehensive list of references is given at the end of the book.
- A summary workbook which relates to a virtual IBL group using a storyboard approach, developed by the author, is included in Appendix 2 (this workbook allows students in postgraduate module *Facilitating IBL* to experience some realistic scenarios).

The approach

The book is presented in four themed parts comprising sixteen chapters sequenced by topic. The logical structure makes it simple to access topics either directly or serially according to preference.

Key features of the chapters

PART I	**Why inquiry-based learning?**
Chapter 1	This is an introductory chapter which gives the background and rationale for the book and the topic and sets the scene for the reader.
Chapter 2	This inquiry-based learning domain chapter shows the many factors of IBL and how to develop and implement an effective IBL approach. It also describes how the IBL student-centred approach differs from a teacher-centred approach.
Chapter 3	This chapter explores the theoretical perspectives of IBL. It provides a point of reference from which to make critical decisions and form a comprehensive appreciation of the theoretical framework relating to IBL.
PART II	**Inquiry-based learning project implementation**
Chapter 4	This chapter considers project implementation. It discusses project structure, management, roles and responsibilities, planning, implementation and evaluation.
Chapter 5	This 'change management' chapter focuses on a change model as it relates to sources of resistance to change and approaches to reduce resistance.
PART III	**Operational practicalities: the subprojects**
Chapters 6–13	These chapters focus on the eight subprojects for implementing the operational aspects of the IBL curriculum. These are: (1) staff development; (2) communication system; (3) classroom compass; (4) practice experience; (5) documentation; (6) electronic resources; (7) library resources; (8) media resources.

PART IV   **By the time tomorrow comes**

Chapters 14–16   'Where are we now' focuses on maintaining momentum. 'Where we are going' describes a curriculum evolution model. A postscript summarizes our experience.

The author hopes that all those who wish to implement a more student-centred curriculum will find something of use to them within these pages.

Acknowledgements

I owe so much to so many. This book is the product of several special people's brains, ears, eyes, hands, energy and time. My gratitude and thanks to the many who helped make this publication a reality. It is impossible to thank you all by name. I am very grateful to Dr Dawn Hillier, Dean, School of Health Care Practice, for her encouragement and faith in me. My sincere thanks are due to many colleagues at the NHS Trusts and APU, especially Hilary Bebb, IBL Evaluator, Maurice Wakeham, Academic Liaison Librarian and Trevor Manning, C&ITS Applications Support Officer. I would also like to acknowledge the contributions of Sue Kersey, Administration Manager, Clare Larcombe, IBL Administrator, and James McKee, IT Technician. My gratitude goes to the IBL facilitators and the pre-registration nursing students who have all shared in the evolution of inquiry-based learning at the university. My gratitude goes also to the postgraduate students in my module *Facilitating Inquiry-Based Learning*: their delight in learning is a constant source of energy – special thanks to one who consented to an extract of her reflections appearing in this book. A big thank you to my family and friends for their interest and patience. Then, the most important thanks of all, to my husband and closest friend, Peter, who – despite the demands of his own work – has supported me in so many meaningful ways. Thanks for always being there for me. This book is dedicated to you.

Why inquiry-based learning?

Chapter 1

Introduction: background

In the past, the belief that psychomotor expertise was all that nurses should aspire to pervaded traditional nurse education and shaped its delivery strategy. The hidden curricular outcome was the socialization of each new intake of students into the order-and-obedience culture of the traditionally trained nurse. Paradoxically, by ignoring higher educational goals and confining its provision to elementary vocational domains, traditional training seems to have engineered its own failure. Student nurses, it appeared, 'were not getting the preparation they needed to take on the job of staff nurses' (Shand 1987: 28). The indoctrination into an authoritarian nursing hierarchy that was embedded in the educational process left the hapless newly qualified staff nurse shorn of almost any analytical capacity and virtually incapable of criticizing, let alone mounting any serious challenge to, the status quo – as Lathlean (1987) observed. These professional inadequacies originated in, or were at least exacerbated by, the traditionally minded schools of nursing as far back as 1986, where Sweeney (1986) saw how teacher-centred approaches stifled critical reasoning and fostered negative attitudes to research, change, and student autonomy.

The United Kingdom Central Council (UKCC) (1986: 33) proposed a realignment of nursing education that would enable it to deliver 'a mature and confident practitioner, willing to accept responsibility, able to think analytically and flexibly, able to recognize a need for further preparation and willing to engage in self development'. Out would go the educationally bankrupt teacher-centred practices that were philosophically opposed to this aim. In would come the student-oriented methods that would signal the end of training by apprenticeship and the advent of the undergraduate student of nursing.

In the mid-1990s, the English National Board for Nursing, Midwifery and Health Visiting (ENB) (1994: 2) called for a more general adoption of those learning approaches that 'enabled [students] to acquire the skill of "learning to learn" and the motivation to continue to do so'. Students should be self-directed individuals, responsible for their own learning during the programme and capable of continuing their education after registration. The realization of this ambition presented a problem to curriculum designers, educators and students, since it entailed a radical departure from traditional teaching/learning practice, with a transfer of knowledge from educator to student. Henceforward what would be taught is the art or skill of learning itself. Students would learn how to learn and gain knowledge directly for themselves without relying on the mediation of educators.

Many nurse educators failed to make the large change in their attitudes and methods that treating students as self-directed adults demands. They persisted with a well-worn teacher-centred approach in spite of its obvious incompatibility with the concepts of personal autonomy, accountability and responsibility that a Department of Health (DoH) (1989) report identified as essential components of contemporary professional nursing practice. Their unwillingness to change, for whatever reason, puts them out of step with the strategic direction chosen by nursing and by nurse education.

Tradition-oriented nurse education institutions have been reproached in a World Health Organization (1993: 3) report because 'Imparting discrete facts and organizing knowledge by discipline simplify the tasks of teachers, but do not necessarily help learners to acquire easily and efficiently the skills they need to address the health problems they are likely to encounter in practice'. Problem-based learning was advanced as an important educational strategy to improve professional education. But despite repeated appeals from regulatory bodies and progressive educationalists like Knowles (1990) to discard the inefficient and ineffective teaching and learning practices of the past, the pedagogical model endures, throwing a long shadow over contemporary nurse education.

Project 2000 was an educational model intended to prepare nursing students to be more able to deal with changing health care demands and provide quality care upon registration. Since it was implemented in 1989, abundant feedback concerning the programme's strengths and weaknesses suggests that practical constraints often meant that the sought after transformation of nurse education has been less radical in operation than planned – especially with regard to its defining attribute, student-centredness. Jowett (1995) and Willis (1996) observed that substantial numbers of nursing students in the common foundation programme were being taught in single large groups. Many students, understandably, find the prospect of asking a question in the presence of a sizeable audience too daunting – and are thereby denied the opportunity to participate in their own learning. Similarly on the other side of the equation, teachers 'have to predominantly lecture to large groups rather than being able to use smaller group methods' (Luker *et al.* 1995). These observations demonstrate that structure tends to determine function. An obvious example is the way in which the physical structure of a lecture hall is designed to enable everyone in the audience to see and hear the lecturer – not each other. Attempts to insert student-centred functions forcibly into structures which are purpose-built to optimize the traditional educational paradigm of teacher-directed lectures and textbooks are fraught with difficulty.

In *Making a Difference* (Department of Health 1999) and *Fitness for Practice* (United Kingdom Central Council 1999), summarized in *Education in Focus* (English National Board for Nursing, Midwifery and Health Visiting 2000), the nursing profession's governing bodies addressed the issue of structure, making radical change in the pre-registration curriculum a key recommendation – along with the development of lifelong learning skills. New structures would support student-centred programmes using new strategies of learning. As Long *et al.* (1999), Gibbon (1998) and Biley and Smith (1998) reported, progressive elements in nurse education were already anticipating these recommendations. A review of the literature shows nurse educators in the United Kingdom implementing one or other of three closely related new learning processes. Though differing somewhat in structure, process steps, terminology and philosophical emphases, these learning strategies draw ideas from the same conceptual well. They are problem-based learning (PBL), enquiry-based learning (EBL) and inquiry-based learning (IBL).

The choice of IBL: a different approach to learning nursing

Anglia Polytechnic University (APU) made the decision to introduce an inquiry-based approach to learning in the pre-registration nursing curriculum in 1998. APU had been moving towards the introduction of a student-centred learning methodology for some time in response to encouragement from statutory and professional bodies – as discussed previously. Progress in this direction quickened when, for instance, nurse practitioners, academics and students began to report that pre-registration nursing students seemed to be experiencing difficulty in transferring knowledge acquired in the theoretical components of the curriculum into the practice area.

The IBL approach introduced in the pre-registration nursing curriculum at APU derives ultimately from the PBL model developed in Canada at McMaster University (Feletti 1993). This had been designed for use in the medical school as a way of overcoming learner passivity and linking theory and practice. Following its conspicuous success at eradicating medical student inertia, PBL radiated from its point of origin to other institutions and professions, including nurse education (Barrows 1996, Rideout and Carpio 2001). IBL was seen to be the best tool that APU could employ to urge students towards active learning and to mount a robust attack on the theory–practice gap.

Although nurse educators enthused over the process of problem-based learning, some found themselves at odds with the label 'problem' (Walton and Matthews 1989). Lest this reservation is thought to be hypercritical, it should be noted that the term is more than just a name. It is integral to the definition of PBL, which considers that every learning experience begins with a problem. There are two reasons why such a premise can only be regarded as unsatisfactory in contemporary nursing. First, it militates against the holistic view of health by implying only problems are of interest, that is, it concentrates attention exclusively on a client's illness rather than examining a client's needs. Second, it implies that discovering a workable solution is equivalent to, or at least as good as, gaining a full understanding – with the consequent danger that new client care strategies might simply be rehashed from existing practices rather than being developed from new research. A more generally acceptable proposition is that every learning experience begins not with a problem but a question. In recognition of this philosophical difference, the alternative designations of enquiry-based learning and inquiry-based learning are tending to find favour in more recent introductions of the methodology – a small but crucial change in emphasis that alters the whole tone of the learning approach when it is implemented.

A further disharmony between PBL and nurse education, which stems one supposes from its origins in medical education, is that it has a diagnostic-like structure – which makes it a fairly formal methodology, unlike IBL which 'starts with fewer assumptions and has broader goals for the students and roles for the teachers' (Feletti 1993: 150). The less rigidly structured, more open IBL approach seems better suited to investigation in clinical circumstances too, where the domains of the individual, society, disease and wellbeing intermingle across fuzzy ill-defined boundaries. It was to exploit this attribute of flexibility that IBL was introduced into the University of Hawaii's School of Nursing in 1992 (Magnussen *et al.* 2000).

By 1993 Feletti felt able to describe a model of IBL that would 'revitalize nursing'. The attractiveness of this model was enhanced by its added functionality – a framework for curriculum planning and evaluation, a number of different learning/teaching approaches to bridge the theory–practice gap, and a template for lifelong learning. It is Feletti's model that has been adapted for use at APU, an educational philosophy and a methodology that are already beginning to revolutionize the activities and aspirations of students, academics and practitioners.

Chapter 2

Inquiry-based learning domains

Defining the IBL model

> IBL is an orientation towards learning that is flexible and open and draws upon the varied skills and resources of faculty and students. Faculty are co-learners who guide and facilitate the student-driven learning experience to achieve the goals of nursing practice. This includes an inter-disciplinary approach to learning and problem-solving, critical thinking and assumption of responsibility by students for their own learning.
>
> (Feletti 1993: 146)

It is evident from the foregoing that some words used in talking about IBL have an import that goes beyond their use in everyday language. To reduce the possibility of confusion or error, a list of the key terms associated with IBL and its implementation are defined here.

Critical thinking The IBL methodology relies on activities like exploration, discussion, analysis and the synthesis of new and old learning, all of which exercise the cluster of investigative and deductive skills that characterize critical thinking. The very act of asking questions is a renunciation of 'things as they are', or, more precisely, a suspension of belief that the situation is really as it is perceived to be and beyond that, a distrust of the habits of mind that shaped that perception. Scepticism about the rightness of the accepted view and a readiness to challenge the status quo are hallmarks of the IBL student and integral to the process of critical thinking and clinical reasoning.

Facilitation The IBL facilitator works in an open partnership with students – encouraging, guiding and supporting their explorations with open-ended questions and by acting as a resource. The facilitator makes a contribution as a learner among learners and is as willing to explore unfamiliar domains of knowledge as any other student.

Flexibility The individuality of students is echoed by differences in the ways in which they prefer to learn. IBL handles individual preferences in learning styles by the deployment of a wide variety of learning methods. The flexibility of provision extends beyond self-directed learning and the IBL tutorial to include, for example, lectures formatted as resource sessions or with content chosen by the students.

Interdisciplinary approach IBL elevates learning with others over learning by oneself. Appropriately differentiated models for collaboration in interdisciplinary and intradisciplinary groups can be employed to promote teamwork (Feletti 1993). The deliberate emphasis on joint learning endeavours seen in IBL represents a radical departure from traditional modes of academic delivery. By combining their disciplines, students, facilitators and practitioners from across the board in the care community are able to fashion a formidable investigatory tool for use in the shared exploration of scenarios.

Openness Openness – intellectual, psychological and emotional – is intrinsic to the IBL approach, where it is a defining attribute of facilitation, a prerequisite for flexibility, and the medium in which the interdisciplinary approach operates. The students 'are open to experience, to new ways of seeing, new ways of being, new ideas and concepts' (Rogers 1980: 350). Openness is a two-way street. It is as much about opening up to others – revealing perhaps unexpected capabilities but also exposing personal limitations – as it is about being open to receive new inputs. Experiencing trust and being trusted promotes self-discipline and responsibility – the requisites of lifelong learning.

Problem-solving Problem-solving is a knowledge dependent activity. The more one knows about the situation described in the scenario, the more able one is to spot the problems in it and find solutions for them. The multifaceted knowledge store of the heterogeneous IBL group greatly increases the effectiveness of this activity.

Use of resources In IBL a resource is anything or anyone that a student has the ingenuity and imagination to identify as a possible source of accurate information, provided only that they have the means to gain legitimate access to that resource. The Web extends the reach of the student far beyond what the library or facilitator may have to offer – although neither of the latter will be neglected. Apart from the advantages that are likely to obtain from the use of wide and varied resources – a greater amount and/or better quality of data – the challenges and rewards of a far-ranging search in themselves can only serve to increase student motivation and sustain a high level of interest.

Responsibility for own learning Obviously, students are wholly responsible for any learning that they do on their own. But they have no less responsibility, to themselves as well as to their fellow learners, when they learn as members of a group – responsibilities that can only be fully discharged when their participation in the shared learning activity is wholehearted and energetic. There can be no responsibility without power. In the IBL tutorial process, students have the power to direct their own learning by constructing their own learning objectives and deciding when, where and by what means – in terms of activities and resources – those objectives will be achieved.

Student-directedness One of the ways in which students demonstrate a greater autonomy and involvement in their education is by asking questions. Since the questions are mostly formulated and posed by students, the students become, by default as well as intention, the ones who mainly direct the process of learning – and by so doing assert their ownership of that process. They do not, of course, have the unlimited freedom of the truly self-taught individual who can follow a line of enquiry wherever fancy dictates. They cannot stray too far from those directions that will lead sooner or later towards the curriculum's outcomes. Nevertheless the IBL approach always 'allow(s) students some choice of how they will learn – either the method itself or the control of the agenda within a given method' (Feletti 1993: 148).

Inquiry-based learning methodology

IBL has been defined as an educational philosophy and a methodology. When adopted as a philosophy, it is implemented at the strategic level – the whole curriculum is redeveloped in accordance with the IBL model as 'an integrated pattern of learning experiences' (Feletti 1993: 149). When employed simply as a learning methodology – in what will otherwise for the most part continue to be a traditional curriculum – it can be implemented either tactically at the modular level or, for a subject area, it could be implemented in an even more piecemeal fashion as just another method of learning – one among several. This last option might arise circumstantially where some academic staff feel inspired to experiment with IBL in a practical way, to evaluate the approach for themselves and/or to demonstrate its capabilities in an unequivocal way to sceptical colleagues.

Where there is a mixed educational offering, i.e. isolated units of IBL embedded in a largely traditional curriculum, problems can be anticipated whenever students cross over from one educational philosophy to a second that is diametrically opposed in every way to the first. For example, as Walton and Matthews (1989) observed, in partial implementations of problem-based learning, student perceptions of traditional assessment may make them take it more seriously and lead them to make less of an effort when working in an isolated IBL module. Then, too, what is regarded as desirable student behaviour could not be more different in each regime and students would have to make a considerable mental adjustment when crossing from one to the other – silent students waiting passively to take notes being as unwelcome in an IBL group as a noisy brainstorming session would be if it broke out in the middle of a carefully prepared lecture.

Moving towards an IBL curriculum little by little is a tempting strategy, especially when confronted with the sheer complexity of transforming and reconciling so many different, and so many difficult, factors, like staff commitment, resource availability, administrative issues. But, given the degree of educational dissonance that exists, it must be doubted whether operating both traditional and IBL approaches in tandem for any length of time is practical from an academic management point of view, or contributes an educational benefit that outweighs the confusion and disruption of the student experience. Barrows (1986: 485) wisely counsels educators 'to decide on desired educational objectives and then select the method that fits best'.

Scenarios

The IBL scenario describes a situation that the students will immediately recognize as being true to life – a situation they might well find themselves in at some time, perhaps have already encountered. Since life is 'full of care' the scenario, to appear realistic, is likely to contain all sorts of individual and societal difficulties and dilemmas, but it will not be simply a concise statement of some clinical problem that can be solved by identifying the correct professional intervention. In IBL the central character does not even need to be a patient/client. The scenario might focus on a community or institutional setting, health educator, the family or, indeed, a student. The scenario's realism helps to ensure 'that the trigger material is relevant, interesting and provokes discussion' (David *et al.* 1999: 4). Obviously it must be carefully authored if it is to address the programme module's core concepts – and achieve its learning outcomes – as well as kickstarting a lively, volatile, constantly evolving student investigation that leaves no stone unturned.

IBL groups

At APU, the distribution of students to groups is determined by specific nursing fields, i.e. adult nursing studies, childhood studies, learning disabilities studies, mental health studies. The basic learning unit in IBL is the small group that cooperatively, with a facilitator, works through scenarios specifically designed to be accurate renditions of reality. When the group meets, it sits in positions that maximize interaction – a circle or semicircle – in a customized IBL room equipped with appropriate learning resources, such as a whiteboard, flipchart, personal computer, television monitor, video player, filing cabinet. The roles of a student group chair and scribe for the tutorials are rotated so that each member has an opportunity to practise team management and support skills, find out how to cope with conflict and learn to use time productively and effectively. Group work develops social as well as intellectual skills, and promotes independence, accountability and self-esteem. The workings of the IBL group exemplify adult learning principles – the skills learned are those needed for continual professional development and a lifetime of learning.

The IBL group cannot be too small because this would mean there was an insufficient variety of background, experience, pre-existing knowledge and learning styles. The richer the mix that students bring to the group, the wider and deeper are the resources the group can call upon – additionally, the energy released by the dynamic interaction of a multitude of disparate elements generates a powerful stimulus to learning. There are differing opinions about how small a group can get and remain viable. The lowest number seen in (PBL) literature is five – see Barrows (1996), Walton and Matthews (1989).

Generally, nursing student intakes are either so large or so frequent that very low student to academic staff ratios are just not feasible. Feletti (1993) makes the additional point that nursing budgets are anyway too constrained to provide customized accommodation for a large number of small groups and, accordingly, recommends a (quite high) lower limit of fifteen. It must be said that this has not been the experience at APU, where, despite an annual intake of about five hundred students, there are ample purpose-fitted IBL rooms to accommodate IBL groups with, typically, a lower limit of ten.

To make best use of limited staff and accommodation resources, could IBL groups be made very large? Unfortunately, overly large groups produce two very different side effects – neither of which are wanted. First, big groups contain greater individual variance and relationship complexity. The group dynamic is therefore more highly-charged and this volatile energy brings with it a greater risk of conflict. Second, and paradoxically, a large group, in effect, de-energizes its weaker members. In a small group everyone is in the front row and cannot help but be drawn in. But in large groups the more vocal and assertive monopolize centre stage, leaving the timid or bashful marginalized – passive observers of the learning of others, instead of active participants in their own.

David *et al.* (1999: 4) sensibly suggest 'the ideal group is one with sufficient numbers to have a reasonable breadth and depth of knowledge but small enough to allow individuals to engage and contribute'. In the University of Hawaii School of Nursing, IBL groups range from eight to ten students (Magnussen *et al.* 2000). In the health schools at APU the IBL groups usually have between ten and fifteen learners.

The IBL tutorial process

In IBL, the tutorial process epitomizes the student-centred, interdisciplinary approach to learning. The IBL tutorial itself closely models the critical reasoning process. Critical reasoning cannot simply be learnt by watching others. This intellectual skill is best mastered by active engagement in group discussion, by argument and counter-argument with one's peers, by self-directed study and the acceptance of responsibility for one's own learning.

The IBL tutorial process begins with group discussion of the scenario, and ends with the group reflecting on what was learned and, importantly, on how it was learned. The process includes periods of self-directed learning as well as working in teams, of library and Web-based research as well as interviewing/consulting individuals with scenario-relevant experience. The five IBL tutorial process steps are described below.

Tutorial process steps

The first session opens with Step 1 (see below), the exploration tutorial – in which the IBL group is for the first time confronted with the scenario that describes the real-life situation they have met to discuss, and for which they must construct the knowledge base needed for a full understanding. Using whatever prior knowledge they can marshal between them, and their imaginations, students employ idea-generating techniques to extract all the meaning they can from the scenario. They isolate issues and identify appropriate concepts to illuminate those issues. In a feedback loop familiar to researchers, the consideration of theoretical understandings generates new insights, leading to the discovery of new areas of concern and interest in the scenario – initiating a further search for yet more theory that might be germane to the exploration.

As the group explores all the implications of the scenario, it bears in mind – and works towards – a number of sub-goals that must be achieved before this initial step can be completed. The students must itemize any issues that they have not been able to resolve in full because the group's pooled prior knowledge proved an inadequate resource. Similarly, there will be some aspects of the scenario about which they know little or nothing. They must decide what questions have to be answered to gain complete understanding. Finally the IBL group must organize all this outstanding learning into discrete tasks, identify what learning resources will be called for, and decide how best to allocate the workload to individuals or small subgroups.

Session 1

Step 1: Exploration tutorial (two hours)

The scenario is presented to the group (realistic, practice-based, open-ended).

Students

- brainstorm concepts and issues extracted from the scenario to find out what is happening:
  - generating broader insights and interests
  - noticing and raising questions
  - exploring their existing knowledge as it relates to the scenario
- define and analyse the nature of the situation to determine gaps in their knowledge
- analyse and prioritize unanswered questions to identify learning issues on aspects of the situation for later exploration (this is the focus of their self-directed studies)
- generate relevant questions about the situation that need to be explored
- decide which learning issues are to be allocated to which individual and identify the resources needed to inquire into the learning issues (the group subdivides the list and works individually or in small groups).

Session 1 continued

Step 2: Self-directed learning

Students

Undertake self-directed learning to gather new additional information prior to Session 2:

- integrate new and prior learning about the situation
- search out answers whenever and by whatever means necessary.

Session 2

Step 3: Review tutorial (two hours)

Students

- present the new information to the group (to share the new information as part of the group process)
- analyse and apply the new information to the scenario situation
- evaluate the effectiveness of the findings of the inquiry
- confirm sources of the new information
- identify unanswered questions to determine new learning issues for further exploration.

NB Step 3 may need to be repeated.

In the educational foreground, the group is learning more about the scenario situation, whilst in the background, often unconsciously, they are learning group skills, like teamworking, committing, collaborating and cooperating. If the scenario, as it often must, touches upon personal issues and emotions that strike a chord with individuals in the group, the students may also find themselves venturing into counselling, caring and mutual support.

The first session culminates in Step 2 (see box above) – where the students pursue their allocated tasks as self-directed learners studying alone or in twos and threes. The outcome each student works towards is the presentation of new findings to the whole group when it reassembles two to three days later for Step 3 – the review tutorial. Within these overarching constraints of final target and timeframe, students make their own choices about goals and objectives, decide what and how they will learn, schedule the workload, select appropriate resources, and determine how they will assess the quality of the results.

Both scheduled and unscheduled time is available to the students for information gathering and analysis. The IBL facilitator's role revolves from resource person to lecturer to guide – to accommodate students' differing learning styles and needs. In addition to purely self-directed learning, student activities in Step 2 may also involve fixed resource lectures, sessions in the skills laboratory, fact-finding visits to clinical and community practice areas, and interviewing professionals and non-professionals who may be able to contribute pertinent input.

The second session is entirely taken up with Step 3 (see p. 13), the review tutorial. The students, or alternatively working subgroups, take turns to impart the new information they have gathered to the whole group, using appropriate presentation skills to communicate effectively what they have found. The sources from which the data was obtained are identified. The group critically appraises the new data, debating any new ideas, and seeing how it fits into what is already known. The scenario situation is revisited to assess how well what has been learned addresses the outstanding issues.

The group may decide that the new information is not valid or it is valid but irrelevant. When data is discarded or discounted in this way, it implies that there is an area of interest or concern in the scenario situation that must be reinvestigated. Or, perhaps, in the critical discussions, fresh concepts or issues may have emerged that need a more detailed appraisal. Or it might simply be the case that when all the new knowledge is put together it is still not enough – areas of interest have been missed or not satisfactorily explained. However it comes about, the group will need to identify any newly emerged issues and determine among themselves how the outstanding items can best be explored. Consequently, it may be necessary to repeat Step 3.

If, after further reiterations of the review tutorial there are still unresolved issues and time is pressing, the group may decide to move on to Step 4, the consolidation tutorial, with what they have, leaving uncompleted lines of inquiry to be pursued informally between the group members. Email as a medium is encouraged for an *ad hoc* group activity like this since it is both time-independent and self-documenting. The students can use the filing cabinet located in each IBL room to file any notes or information for review or follow-up at a later date.

Session 3

Step 4: Consolidation tutorial (two hours)

Students

- develop an action plan focusing on the scenario situation, stating the rationale for the action
- present the action plan to the group for discussion and review.

Session 4

Step 5: Plenary tutorial (two hours)

Students

- reflect on individual and group learning with the facilitator – on changes resulting from the learning experiences
- identify further learning needs.

The third session comprises Step 4 (see p. 14), the consolidation tutorial. Once the students are satisfied that they have an understanding of the salient features of the situation described in the scenario, they can operationalize what they have learned. There is a range of possibilities about how action plans to meet the needs of the situation can be developed. Each individual student or subgroup may create a rationalized action plan for the issue they researched. If some areas of interest are closely related then the associated issues may be clumped and a composite action plan developed for them by those involved in their exploration. Or the whole IBL group might decide that the optimal approach would be for them all to come together to produce an integrated action plan that addresses each of the concerns raised in the scenario.

The last session is the plenary tutorial, Step 5 (see above) – in which students look back on their learning experience metacognitively. They critically review how the learning process worked for them, as individuals and as a group. Were they able to plan and implement learning in the way they wished? Were there obstacles to learning, like a lack of skill, resources or time, that compromised their plans? How, on reflection, could they have identified those obstacles in time to find ways round them? In short: what went right, what went wrong and why? As individuals and as a group, how has the experience already changed them, and what else should they change?

Roles and responsibilities within the tutorial process

Student

In the IBL curriculum, learners are both product and process, customer and stakeholder, students who teach themselves. That IBL students are responsible for, and have real control of, their learning is nowhere made more apparent than in the tutorial process. In traditional modes of teaching and learning, the teacher directed the business of the class, choosing, for instance, who shall speak and for how long. And, more subtly, the teacher – by monopolizing the whiteboard and what was written on it – chose what was to be heard and recorded as 'learned'.

In IBL these two cornerstones of teacher power, the functions of chairperson and scribe, are exercised by students. Chair and scribe are elected by the group as a preliminary to exploring the scenario.

The chair helps the group to work effectively and efficiently through the scenario using the tutorial process and, for example, reminding potential transgressors of the agreed ground rules, using their casting vote to resolve amicable disagreement and checking with the facilitator acting as an independent monitor of the group's workings with regard to relevance, accuracy and completeness. The chair also coordinates the group's allocation of learning issues among its members.

The scribe is the group's minute-taker. As the group works through the scenario – generating ideas, agreeing items of interest and significance, identifying activities and tasks, making plans – the scribe maintains an open public record on flipchart and/or whiteboard for later transcription and distribution to group members.

The roles of chair and scribe are inclusively rotated through the whole group so that every student gets an opportunity to play each part. As well as the immediate benefits of acquiring and practising managerial and people skills in the execution of their role, the chair and scribe gain in other ways. Their formal office disengages them slightly from their peers, allowing them an external perspective on the learning process – like the facilitator's. This is a metacognitive experience since they become observers of the learning process – seeing from the outside how it's done – at the same time as they are participants in it. The other metalearning gain is that the external function they perform for the group is one that when they come to study alone, they must perform for themselves. For example, the scribe learns the importance of capturing ideas and insights immediately and of drawing up formal plans of action. These skills and understandings gained in practice, once they are internalized by the student, will greatly enhance self-directed learning.

Facilitator

The facilitator's first task is to introduce the scenario to the whole IBL group. From that point onward, the facilitator retires from the limelight and becomes the group's guide, not its instructor. The role is supportive and advisory in nature. The facilitator is not present to provide answers (Schwartz *et al.* 2001), but to ask questions – questions that broaden the group's perspective and encourage the group members to ask more relevant, more pointed, questions themselves. Better indeed if the facilitator is not a subject expert and does not even know the answers – spoon-feeding learners from the facilitator's store of knowledge derails the whole tutorial process (Engle 1998).

The facilitator does need to be an expert in social dynamics, able to foster teamwork and cooperation – so that the group can enjoy the synergic benefits that come from active collaboration – and be equally adept at defusing any conflict that might arise as a consequence of the close association of diverse, perhaps antagonistic, personalities.

Operational guidelines for the facilitator in the tutorial process

Exploration tutorial: guidelines for facilitators

- Present the scenario as a stimulus to the students. Encourage the students to identify the issues in the scenario sentence by sentence.
- Encourage students through active questioning to discuss the scenario in relation to their previous knowledge and experience.
- Encourage students to brainstorm their ideas in relation to the nature and causes of the situation.
- Encourage students critically to analyse the situation, to identify gaps in their knowledge (questioning methods based on, for example, What? Why? When? Who? How?).
- Help them to identify their learning needs through questioning.
- Encourage them to investigate what they need to learn further.

NB Try not to take over the session with own experiences, stories or reflections.

Review tutorial: guidelines for facilitators

- Encourage students to make their presentation interesting and stimulating, for example guided imagery, role play, providing handouts, etc.
- Agree a set time for students' presentation.
- Encourage students to apply the new information gained to the initial scenario.

Consolidation tutorial: guidelines for facilitators

- Encourage students to develop their action plan and present it to the group.
- Participate in the group discussion. Use active questioning methods to clarify the various areas of the action plan.

Plenary session: guidelines for facilitators

- Encourage students to reflect on the learning process.
- Review the achievement of the learning outcomes.

Resource session

Feletti's (1993) model allows for student activities that are tutor, as well as student, instigated. These are learning and teaching methods that are additional to, and supportive of, the tutorial process, such as lectures, seminars and skills laboratory demonstrations. The value of non-exclusivity in the IBL methodology is twofold. First, it makes it possible for the IBL curriculum to cater for the full range of student learning style preferences. Second, provided they are designed with a specific educational purpose in mind, other methods of learning can be very effective. The broad stroke lecture delivered to 'cover a subject' is rightly condemned (Walton and Matthews 1989: 552), but the lecture given by an expert as a masterclass can be the approach of choice where the knowledge domain is cutting edge or especially abstruse.

At APU, there are opportunities during the one-year foundation programme for shared learning between different field specific groups in resource sessions and the skills laboratory.

Conclusion

The concepts and techniques of IBL have been described in this chapter as they are understood, and as they have been deployed, in the pre-registration nursing programme at APU. The implementation of IBL philosophy and methodology at APU will differ subtly, perhaps markedly, from implementations at other educational institutions. IBL is nothing if not flexible so its orientation is likely to be influenced by the local academic-service culture as well as by the peculiarities of the physical environment in which it has been operationalized. However, we do not feel that we have strayed far from the basic Feletti model and believe that if we continue as we have started our students will complete the programme demonstrating all the desirable learning outcomes that the IBL approach promises.

Chapter 3

Theoretical perspectives of inquiry-based learning

Introduction

The salient features of IBL – student autonomy, active learning with understanding, clinical reasoning, collaboration in a social context – indicate that it is ideologically closely related to constructivism, learning how to learn, metalearning and emancipatory learning. A brief examination of these other theoretical perspectives provides useful insights into the origins and nature of IBL and how it might be implemented.

Constructivism

Constructivism starts with the premise that knowledge cannot be transferred from one person to another. 'New knowledge is "constructed" . . . from within individuals through experience' (Hendry *et al.* 1999: 359). For the constructivist, knowledge is an amalgam of understandings commingled in a dynamic interaction between the learner's existing knowledge – accumulated by living through and making sense of a multitude of actual happenings in the past – and the present learning experience. The present learning experience must be lived through too – constructivism 'is about active engagement with the task whether working individually or collaboratively with others' (Ryan 1998: 128). The learning task of necessity should be real, or at least realistic, using actual data from primary sources so as to expose the student to pure information that has not been contaminated or denatured by being pre-processed in the minds of lecturers or the authors of texts.

Each individual's existing knowledge by these definitions is a unique personal mix. Accordingly, the students comprising an IBL group will come to the learning situation from as many different directions, and in as many different states of readiness to learn, as there are students in the group. Student autonomy in these circumstances is a given – since each student must find their own way in the search for meaning.

These notions of the primacy of student-centredness stand in diametrical opposition to those which animate traditional teaching and learning: where lectures and textbooks are media for the passive transfer of knowledge from teacher to class;

where the same content is delivered at the same time to all students; and where a bid for learning autonomy by a student is regarded as a disruptive breach of classroom discipline.

Constructivist ideas have contributed important conceptual strands to inquiry-based learning. Constructing knowledge and student individuality and autonomy dominate IBL methodology. The starting point for the IBL student group is a scenario that presents a true-to-life work situation. Students contribute insights and understandings from their own individual store of uniquely configured knowledge, which means the group is exposed to alternative views, to discrepancies and inconsistencies. The students must reconcile alternatives, resolve differences, whilst they search for new data – ideally from primary sources – to add to the old, from which individually and together they generate possible explanations. Students construct their own knowledge. In effect, knowledge is the emergent product of the synthesis of brainstorming, discussion and reflection on what is known and what has been discovered. Although each student is alone responsible for their learning, IBL is at every step a social activity. 'Collaborative groups are important because we can test our own understanding and examine the understanding of others as a mechanism for enriching, interweaving, and expanding out understanding of particular issues of phenomena' (Savery and Duffy 1995: 32).

The students work as a group with the encouragement of the IBL facilitator. The meaning of the term 'facilitator' in IBL is similar to its use in constructivist education where 'Teaching cannot take center stage' (Peters 2000: 168) and the defined role of the educator is to guide rather than direct, and to support rather than lead, student learning. This is an approach to education that, in accordance with androgogic philosophy, advances self-directed and lifelong learning.

Learning how to learn

'Learning how to learn involves possessing, or acquiring, the knowledge and skill to learn effectively in whatever situation one encounters' (Smith 1983: 19). Throughout life humans have to learn to adapt to changing circumstances. Often change occurs gradually, giving ample time for trial-and-error learning of the new knowledge and skills that are needed. But students working through an intensive programme of study can rarely afford the luxury of random learning behaviour. They need a planned learning strategy to maximize insights and minimize unproductive effort. 'One of the most commonly stated views about higher education is that the most important thing we can achieve for our students is to help them to "learn how to learn"' (Ross 1995: 177).

Learning how to learn is sometimes thought to involve little more than the building up of a modest repertoire of practical study techniques, such as note-taking or speed-reading. Such underrating may have undesirable educational consequences. The learner may neglect to use what was learned and thereby throw away what might have become golden keys to knowledge. Worse, ironically, the student may continue to apply the methods slavishly – 'The increased use of study skills programmes concentrating solely on techniques . . . may be detrimental to the development of more complex conceptions' (Martin and Ramsden 1987: 157). This is a familiar educational dead end. The practical approach when it is unstructured and uninformed by theory does not yield deep understandings, only shallow and poorly connected facts.

The difference between an assortment of study skills and a full-blown learning how to learn strategy is that the latter 'can meet the lifelong need to adapt to contemporary knowledge, challenges and problems they [students] will encounter in the future' (Glasgow 1997: 35). Using similar self-directed learning behaviours and procedures to those found in the IBL model, students are confronted with relevant concepts and issues in the form of a scenario. Before selecting appropriate learning resources, they identify which issues to pursue, what outcomes are wanted and what level of motivation exists to achieve those outcomes – so that the effort in achieving each outcome is proportionate to its value. The findings of their researches in the learning situation are formally presented to others. This is a more thoughtful and deliberate way to gain knowledge and understanding – one that has a greater chance of success than using superficial and untargeted study skills, because it is based on 'engagement with the material, with others, and with the self' (Anderson 1992: 239).

Simple study skills are an assemblage of rote learned 'how to' procedures that can be categorized as essentially pedagogical in their educational orientation. In many educational programmes study skills are presented once in a pre-course induction, never to be mentioned again. The self-directing, critical thinking and problem-solving features of 'learning how to learn' clearly designate it as andro-gogical – just as with IBL. Indeed 'The idea of learning how to learn can be stressed as a condition for optimum adult learning and taught as such' (Smith 1983: 30). Its concepts should be addressed at the start of programmes for new students and continually promoted thereafter to develop competent and motivated learners – initiating 'a lifelong process by means of which students can continue to build on the learning that takes place in the course' (Alavi and Cook 1995: 126).

Metalearning

Metalearning starts when the student becomes aware of how they learn how to learn,

> when learning reaches a special stage: when the Seeker realizes that he is acquiring knowledge in a range beyond 'seeking' and 'finding', or 'being sought'.
>
> (Pahlawan-i-Zaif, cited by Shah 1990: 249)

Metacognition is that field of scientific inquiry that concerns itself with how much self-knowledge learners have about their cognitive processes and what effect that knowledge has on their learning. Metalearning 'is a subprocess of metacognition

. . . that refers specifically to learning and study processes in institutional settings, and more particularly to students' awareness of their motives, and control over their strategy selection and deployment' (Biggs 1985: 192). Metalearning is a self-referential activity in which the student's mind reflects upon its own intellectual functioning to determine what strengths and weaknesses in cognitive capability need to be taken into account when approaching a learning task. This self-referring dimension together with the importance that is given to understanding abstract concepts of mentality – both key components of the IBL tutorial process – serve to distinguish metalearning from learning how to learn strategies, where theoretical considerations are more directly linked to the practicalities of acquiring and deploying study skills.

In metalearning, the function of experiential information from the external environment is to prompt a review and possible reformation of the internal rules and assumptions that govern the student's customary interactions with the outside world. This is more in keeping with androgogic precepts of student autonomy. The student who sees the 'situation clearly and who freely takes responsibility for that situation is a very different person from the one who is simply in the grip of outside circumstances' (Rogers 1983: 278). The educator's responsibility in IBL shifts away from directing students through a programme of learning experiences. It becomes centred rather on helping students to develop their metacognitive awareness – since 'Learning is quicker when students possess self-monitoring skills generally referred to as metacognition' (Gijselaers 1996: 15).

Freire (1972: 15) coined the word 'conscientization' to describe how growing self-awareness of the innermost workings of their intellects encourages students to challenge preconceptions, ingrained attitudes and habitual patterns of living that put a fence around what it is possible to learn, and curb intellectual growth. The consequent discovery and adoption of more powerful, alternative, modes of thinking enables students to become engaged with ever more complex structures of knowledge.

There is a danger that the truly transforming potential of this process of 'conscientious' review and questioning may not be grasped. 'If students do not see the point . . . or are unmotivated to commit themselves to the deeper involvement in learning that this requires, they will treat it as just another cognitive, not a metacognitive, activity' (Biggs 1985: 209). To avoid 'short-changing' students in this way, would-be IBL educators need vigorously to employ those highly compatible androgogic principles – empowerment and encouragement of self-direction – to incite the sort of deep processing that elevates understanding over surface memory and fuels the synthesis of new ideas. As Bruning, Schrow and Ronning (1995 cited by Gijselaers 1996: 15) suggest, the development of metacognitive learning skills in students by providing appropriate learning experience is key to their educational progress. Or, more poetically,

'Teach me how to learn and what to study'. And, even before that: 'Let me really wish to learn how to learn, as a true aspiration, not simply in self-pretence'.

(Khwaja Ali Ramitani, cited by Shah 1990: 292)

Emancipatory learning

Despite Milligan's (1999) reservations about the extent to which emancipatory potentials can be fully realized in PBL, a review of the literature gives some assurance that the emancipatory approach to learning provides a plausible theoretical basis for IBL.

The emancipatory approach is one of the three paths, or levels, to gaining knowledge contained in a model of dominance-free communication created by Habermas (1978). The least effective path, at the lowest level in the model, is technical learning – which equates to surface learning – where the intention is merely to reproduce facts. The highest and most effective level is 'Emancipatory learning . . . the most in-depth, the most comprehensive form of knowing' (Apps 1988: 119). Between these two lies practical learning, a deep approach motivated by the desire to understand the meaning of things. 'The least familiar of the three areas or domains, the emancipatory, is of particular interest to educators' (Mezirow 1983: 124), mainly because it addresses explicitly the social–cultural–individual matrix in which the learning process is embedded.

In traditional education, the intrinsic and extrinsic factors that influence learning are either ignored as irrelevant or, if thought to be relevant, stipulated and wholly controlled by those in authority. Traditional education is a product-driven strategy where the ends are more important than the means. Progressive education strives to reduce the impact of any negative external factors and encourage the development of positive internal factors, in the expectation that by so optimizing student learning, satisfactory educational outcomes will in due course be obtained. It is a process-driven strategy where the means are just as important as, perhaps in some ways more important than, the ends. The emancipatory approach goes beyond these to tackle the social–cultural–individual complex head-on:

> Emancipatory learning has as its purpose the freeing of people from the personal, institutional, or environmental forces that may prevent them from seeing new perspectives for their lives, from attaining broader and deeper goals in their lives, from gaining control over their lives and their communities beyond.
>
> (Apps 1988: 118)

Here any formal educational outcomes are subsumed in an all-enveloping internal and external revolutionary process of learning-to-live and living-to-learn, in which the means become the ends.

In IBL, the first steps towards dominance-free communication are taken when students cultivate a heightened sense of critical awareness about the nature and origin of various impediments that lie in the path of their learning. These internal or external obstructions may be repressive or restrictive in their action, or may stem from simple ignorance. Emancipation comes about when IBL students use their newly developed critical perspective to free themselves from the chains, whether conceptual or physical, that previously impeded and distorted their intellectual growth.

Adult education theorists, such as Mezirow (1983), Brookfield (1986, 1993) and Hart (1985) agree that gaining a discerning critical perspective is a prerequisite for student empowerment. Indeed Mezirow (1983: 125), building on Habermas (1978) and Freire (1972), claims 'perspective transformation' is the defining characteristic of adult education since it is 'the learning process by which adults come to recognize their culturally induced dependency roles and relationships and the reasons for them and take action to overcome them'. Students who are unable to break free of the initial state of childish dependency never become fully self-reflecting adults. Their selfhood is defined by others – they are passive objects in their own existences. 'Self-reflection is . . . emancipation, comprehension, and liberation from dogmatic dependence' (Habermas 1978: 208). With intensified self-reflection, liberating concepts and understandings are integrated into the maturing self, whilst old restricting beliefs and assumptions are repudiated. 'Emancipatory learning integrates a variety of points of view, it brings together opposing positions, it examines the past and the present, it includes knowledge from a wide sweep of disciplines and, very importantly, it includes one's own views and feelings' (Apps 1985: 152) – a summary of defining characteristics that can be applied equally well to IBL.

Clearly it would be too optimistic to expect the self-sufficient functionality looked for in the contemporary nurse to be cultivated in bureaucratic surroundings, using traditional modes of instruction that reinforce the status quo. What is called for are 'methods and techniques which involve the individual most deeply in self-directed inquiry' (Knowles 1983: 68). For emancipatory learning, students may need to be helped to recognize how limiting an unquestioning acceptance of familiar trains of thought can be. This almost certainly requires an open, yet supportive, learning environment in which alternative strategies can be examined and actively tested. Indeed according to Knowles' (1990) androgogic arguments, providing appropriate educational conditions may be all that is needed since adults are naturally self-directed in their learning. More modestly, Garrigan (1997) proposes a degree of facilitation and support to help students towards independence, to a recognition of their learner status, and an acceptance that they are responsible for their own learning.

> I have learned what I have learned only after my teachers had freed me of the habit of attaching myself to what I regard as teachers and teachings.
> (Zikira ibn El-Yusufi, cited by Shah 1990: 291)

Eclectic model for IBL

Some major learning approaches have been brought together in the eclectic model to facilitate critical analysis and offer new insights into IBL.

A variety of constructs has been identified to categorize student approaches to learning. The best-known of these are the surface and deep approaches. These form the opposing dimensions of a bipolar model delineating a philosophical continuum in which behaviouristic concepts inform the 'surface' dimension, and some human-istic concepts inform the 'deep'. Although the emancipatory approach discussed earlier shares many features with deep learning, there are discrepancies. Crucially, deep learning is centred on the learning task, at least in Marton and Säljö's (1976) perspective. In their interpretation, it is the relative difficulty of the learning task that prompts the student to choose an appropriate learning approach. The ideological conflict in Marton and Säljö's deep learning theory is resolved to some extent by Biggs' (1985) formulation that looks beyond the learning task to emphasize the importance of the student's personal motivations and feelings. Biggs' intrinsically motivated version of deep learning has more in common with the humanistic philosophy of living that animates the emancipatory approach and thus IBL.

The range of constructs employed to promote IBL has drawn from a diversity of domains concerned with study and cognition, motivation and behaviour, humanism and autonomy, and experience, resulting in a conceptual and ideological assortment. Readily observable correspondences and affinities in these constructs make it possible to devise a simple model, pulling together what has already been done, to test some common assumptions about how IBL students learn how to learn.

The 'eclectic' model, adapted from Cleverly (1995), is a consolidated conceptual framework for considering metalearning (see Figure 3.1). Where there are overlaps in the contributing theories, their redundant features have been removed to limit the complexity of the model. The design intention is that the remaining core features should associate synergistically in the model – offering a representative and easy-to-survey inventory of the characteristics and effects of the selected approaches.

On the far left of the model are listed some typical teaching/learning strategies. These are loosely clustered according to conceptual allegiance and degree of identification with certain ways of learning. The selection is illustrative, intended for discussion and argument, not a definitive list of all possible strategies. The strategies are shown feeding into the approaches to learning, each of which occupies its own box in the middle of the model. Certain teaching/learning strategies, like rote learning, have an exclusive one-to-one relationship with the surface approach. These are clustered at the top of the left-hand column. Other strategies, like critical analysis, that are wholly alien to surface learning but may be compatible with either, or both, the deep and emancipatory approaches, are gathered below. The three complementary approaches to learning are shown: namely, surface, deep and emancipatory.

Ramsden and Entwistle (1981) and Biggs (1978) made reference to additional dimensions, respectively 'achieving' and 'internalising'. These are not really discrete approaches in their own right but ways in which the elementary surface and deep approaches are operationalized or integrated. The emancipatory approach by contrast is a fully developed pathway to knowledge that stands on an equal footing with the other two basic approaches, earning its place in the eclectic model.

To the right of the model are the expected student outcomes of the various approaches to learning. Just as the surface approach has its own exclusive teaching/learning strategies, so too it has unique outcomes – although retention of facts is

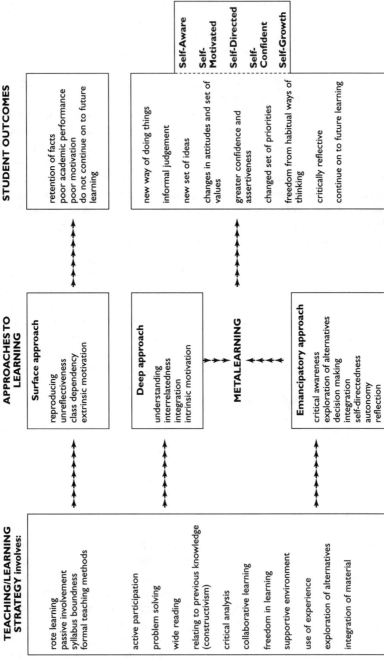

Figure 3.1 Eclectic model of metalearning

TEACHING/LEARNING STRATEGY involves:

rote learning
passive involvement
syllabus boundness
formal teaching methods

active participation
problem solving
wide reading
relating to previous knowledge (constructivism)
critical analysis
collaborative learning
freedom in learning
supportive environment
use of experience
exploration of alternatives
integration of material

APPROACHES TO LEARNING

Surface approach

reproducing
unreflectiveness
class dependency
extrinsic motivation

Deep approach

understanding
interrelatedness
integration
intrinsic motivation

METALEARNING

Emancipatory approach

critical awareness
exploration of alternatives
decision making
integration
self-directedness
autonomy
reflection

STUDENT OUTCOMES

retention of facts
poor academic performance
poor motivation
do not continue on to future learning

new way of doing things
informal judgement
new set of ideas
changes in attitudes and set of values
greater confidence and assertiveness
changed set of priorities
freedom from habitual ways of thinking
critically reflective
continue on to future learning

Self-Aware

Self-Motivated

Self-Directed

Self-Confident

Self-Growth

EMANCIPATORY LEARNING GOALS	EMANCIPATORY LEARNING APPROACHES	IBL TUTORIAL PROCESS STEPS
To become critically aware	Notice changes, differences. Try to recognize problems by: • brainstorming • questioning, examining • analysing • challenging	**Step 1** Exploration tutorial • explore existing knowledge relating to the scenario to find out what is happening and identify learning issues
To explore alternatives	Investigate new ideas and methods of doing things, drawing widely from other disciplines, experiences and feelings	**Step 2** Self-directed learning • research • collect new additional information
To achieve integration	Incorporate novel ideas with old to create new ways of thinking: • reconcile opposing views • explore past experience from present perspective	**Step 3** Review tutorial • analyse and apply the new information to the situation being explored
To implement change	• implement new ideas and approaches • begin to make changes • plan for the future	**Step 4** Consolidation tutorial • develop an action plan
To reflect and evaluate	• review previous steps/goals to gain new awareness • identify further learning needs	**Step 5** Plenary tutorial • review individual and group learning

Figure 3.2 Conceptual framework for understanding the IBL process

the only one of these that could have the remotest academic appeal. The lower box shows the much more desirable outcomes that can be obtained when the educationally superior teaching/learning strategies associated with the deep and emancipatory approaches are utilized. The latter approaches are united by metalearning and constructivism, modes of cognition that are the gateway to higher levels of learning and more advanced states of individual intellectual, emotional and, perhaps, spiritual freedom.

Although it might be argued that a truly emancipated student could freely choose to follow the strategies and approaches that lead to the poor outcomes depicted in the upper right-hand box, it seems unlikely that a student could practise surface learning and remain autonomous. The constant state of heightened self-awareness needed to sustain metalearning would not, it is felt, survive any extended contact with the passivity, unreflectiveness and dependency of surface learning.

Conceptual framework

The conceptual framework that provides IBL with its operational basis is founded upon the goals and strategies of emancipatory learning (see Figure 3.2). Drawing from the work of Apps (1988) and Mezirow (1991), the conceptual framework can be described as follows:

1   The first step towards students' freedom from dependency is taken when students cultivate a heightened sense of critical awareness about their experiences and possibilities. Emancipation comes about when students use their newly developed critical perspective to free themselves from dependencies that previously impeded and distorted their intellectual growth. Promoting such a critical perspective is a prerequisite for student empowerment.

2   The search for knowledge from a wide range of sources, and students' views, experiences and feelings will provide students with a comprehensive perspective. Emancipatory learning activities will encourage and support students in the development of knowledge, participation in research and self-directedness that are associated with adult education.

3   Achieving an effective integration of knowledge, experience and feelings will resolve the contradictions that would otherwise tend to inhibit the constructivist objective of the unification of new learning and prior knowledge. The ready incorporation of new learning into already well-established ways of learning, knowledge or practice will enable students to develop a fully integrated attitude to life that is especially significant for the undergraduate nurse who must follow academic and vocational paths at the same time.

4   Theory is not learned effectively in isolation from practice. Students must relate theory to practice by making operational use of newly acquired ideas and approaches. The assumption is that students are not passive but active individuals who are able to learn and practise in unison.

5   Re-examination of learning may lead to new awakenings and reflective changes in the students' original understandings, or may move students into a new cycle of reflection. Students will be enabled to evaluate the probable effectiveness of their practice.

The conceptual framework enables students to analyse, reflect upon, and gain understandings of previous life experiences in the light of new knowledge.

Conclusion

In conclusion, some theoretical perspectives and approaches have been summarized and their joint contribution to the philosophy and process of IBL discussed. The eclectic model and conceptual framework, as described above, could be useful guides for educators and students.

The structure of the eclectic model graphically illustrates the kinds of teaching/ learning strategies that are characteristic of different approaches and the student outcomes expected from them. The poor quality student outcomes are linked to those strategies usually regarded as the mainstay of training. The more desirable student outcomes of IBL are associated with progressive educational strategies and metalearning constructivist approaches.

Finally, the conceptual framework of IBL provides the process by which critically reflective students will be able to make nursing knowledge and practice their own through the active integration of theoretical concepts with practice. Student academic progression is supported and enhanced by a corresponding movement of students towards self-awareness and intellectual emancipation.

Part II

Inquiry-based learning project implementation

Chapter 4

The implementation project

Introduction

We abstracted the IBL philosophy and methodology out of books and journals and built from them and our experience, the multitude of physical processes and procedures that make up the functionality of an integrated whole curriculum – a curriculum that was going to be used by hundreds of staff and thousands of students in the real world. A truly awesome task, both in prospect and subsequently in actual practice. Fortunately, there is a set of tried and tested tools and techniques available for use in implementing large-scale and complex systems that greatly increase the likelihood of a successful outcome, namely, project management – an approach which 'provides structure, focus, flexibility and control in the pursuit of results' (Bruce and Langdon 2000: 6).

This chapter gives an account of how the IBL implementation project was managed at Anglia Polytechnic University (APU) that is sufficiently complete to inform and guide others with concerns and responsibilities in similar undertakings. Some of the terms used in the following discussion are given at the end of this chapter. More detailed descriptions of the implementation are given, subproject by subproject, in later chapters.

Project management considerations

Every project takes place in a unique set of circumstances and for that reason every project is unique. But not unique in every way – most projects can be broken down into basic components so similar they are normally susceptible to the same general management approach. For example, they can usually be simplified by splitting the elements that need to be managed into two main divisions: the human resource, and the task itself.

Looking at the human resource directly involved in the APU implementation: first, the IBL coordinator is a full-time academic line manager assigned to the IBL implementation. Like the IBL coordinator, all those others contributing to the project also had full-time commitments elsewhere – there were no project members who worked on the IBL project and nothing else. Second, 'a project is likely to involve activities that extend beyond [the project manager's] immediate depart-ment' (Thomsett 2002: 7) – and in the implementation of a whole curriculum that describes most activities. Nevertheless, the IBL coordinator did not have direct control over project members. It might be thought that it would be especially difficult to bring the implementation of a major project to a successful conclusion using a team of 'spare-timers' and relying on the power of persuasion rather than the force of authority. This is to reckon without the initial impetus given by the unreserved support of senior management, who gave an unequivocal message that project-related matters were to be given high priority by all staff. A more powerful motivation soon overtook that first top-down spur to action as the interest and enthusiasm of many staff picked up with increasing awareness of the benefits that IBL might bring – soon rising to a self-sustaining level of commitment and involvement.

The task component of a project is all those activities that the human resource engages in together with the end products of those activities. In the classic project management definition, these end products must be:

- produced within an agreed timescale
- produced within an agreed cost budget
- satisfactory to users.

Each of these intended outcomes lies in the future, so there is necessarily a degree of doubt attached to whether they can be achieved or not. There is a risk that the project will run out of time, or money, or that after it is implemented it will not match up to the expectations of users. Contingencies will be needed to offset those risks which are estimated to be most likely to occur and/or have the greatest potential for causing damage: extra time built into the schedule in case some activities take longer than estimated; an emergency fund for cost overruns; a fallback strategy if implementation should fail, such as a partial implementation of those parts that work, or an orderly reversion to the existing system.

The human resource and the project activities are brought together in the main project processes of:

- planning what, when, where, how and by whom everything is to be done
- implementing: undertaking the planned activities and producing the intended outputs in accordance with the agreed schedule
- evaluating the success or failure of the IBL implementation in achieving the project goals.

Organizational structure

> A project organization is a temporary organization designed to achieve specific results by using teams of specialists from different functional areas within the organization. The team focuses all of its energies and skills on the assigned project.
>
> (Gordon *et al.* 1990: 256)

The project structure adopted to manage the IBL curriculum implementation is shown in Figure 4.1.

The IBL Curriculum Management Group (CMG) was formed following validation of the IBL curriculum. It is a partnership between APU and Health Service Providers. Membership includes:

*   local National Health Service (NHS) hospital trusts, health authorities and primary care groups
*   Workforce Development Confederation
*   IBL evaluator
*   pre-registration nursing programme field leaders
*   foundation programme coordinator.

Others attend by invitation when relevant as co-opted members, for example, the librarian, practice placements manager and health business centre representative.

The IBL coordinator chairs the group meetings – which are held monthly. The group's function is project planning and development and operational management for implementation and evaluation of the curriculum. It provides a central point of liaison, especially for the specialist project teams.

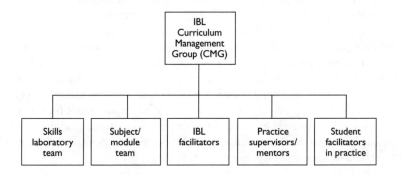

Figure 4.1 IBL project organizational structure

The IBL coordinator

In its pre-implementation phase, the IBL coordinator functions as the project manager, with authority and responsibility for the planning and development of the operational aspects of the IBL curriculum and its successful implementation in the pre-registration nursing programme. Post-implementation, there is a change of emphasis in the role and the IBL coordinator functions as a general manager with authority and responsibility for the operational aspects of the IBL curriculum.

Administration assistance

The administrative staff's technical contribution is vital. In recognition of this, and to add value to their contribution to the project, it makes a great deal of sense to provide all administrative staff with a comprehensive orientation to inquiry-based learning.

An administrative staff dedicated full-time to the project, who is committed and who possesses the requisite skills in communication, word processing and desk-top publishing, is indispensable, particularly where the project is large, the timescales pressing, and all documentation is new. The proactive, self-initiating role of the IBL administrator fulfils three important requirements: gathering and distributing management information; the quality control of documents; and the role of liaison with internal and external personnel.

Every manager has five basic ways of processing information: documents, telephone, scheduled meetings, unscheduled meetings and observational tours. The IBL coordinator, like any manager, is highly reliant on the verbal/face-to-face ways of communicating for timely information (and the opportunity to monitor morale and enthuse project team members). At meetings it is essential that the IBL administrator records the action points agreed verbally in hard copy for imme-diate distribution to all parties. Without hard copy as reference and reminder, the momentum of, and commitment to, the project soon evaporates.

The second important function of the IBL administrator is, with the IBL coordinator, ensuring that documents in the IBL pre-registration nursing curriculum conform to certain standards. One reason for standardization is to promote the IBL house style – to raise the project's profile and build user loyalty. Another reason is to make sure that the quality of presentation and content are consistent throughout the IBL curriculum: to make documents more easily accessible and to prevent some users being disadvantaged because, for example, their module guides are not as informative as those of other modules. A third important function is the maintenance of a network of contacts to gather information for the project.

Overall purpose and structure of project

The purpose of the project was to implement IBL in the context of a modular system. The operational areas that fell within the broad remit of the project were divided into eight subprojects. This division had the dual merit that it made what was a very large project less unwieldy and each subproject could be scheduled for development as a separate entity. The subprojects were:

1   Staff development
2   Communication system
3   Classroom compass
4   Practice experience
5   Documentation
6   Electronic resources
7   Library resources
8   Media resources.

Project planning stage

Time spent in planning is rarely time wasted. Implementation is quicker and smoother when problems have been anticipated and nullified at the planning stage. A further consideration is that implementation is not only a public activity but one that attracts a great deal of attention from stakeholders and users – better by far to discover and correct mistakes in the planning meetings.

To make it more manageable, the whole planning process was initially broken down into five planning steps – adapted from Bruce and Langdon (2000). The steps are shown in Figure 4.2.

In Step 1 and Step 2 the purpose of the project is expanded and restated as specific goals. These are the outcomes that the project is intended to achieve. They cover the specific areas of change with which the project is concerned. The goals are:

1   Prepare academic and practice staff for their new role
2   Improve communication with staff and students
3   Create a learning environment conducive to IBL philosophy
4   Develop appropriate practice experience for students
5   Provide information related to the programme
6   Prepare for access to IT systems
7   Provide access to appropriate learning material
8   Provide quality support for media and equipment.

Step 3 is concerned with making decisions about ways and means, and determining priorities: what activities must be undertaken , and how we use the resources at our command, to achieve the goals that have been identified in Step 2 – within agreed limits of time and cost. It is often observed that there is more than one way to achieve a goal. The challenge for the project coordinator is to find the one way that leads to the goal with the most speed, the least effort and the least risk – the optimal route to success.

In practice the number of alternative ways to reach the project goals can be compromised by circumstances:

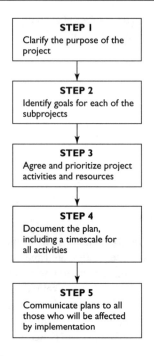

Figure 4.2 IBL project planning process steps

- Resource constraints, especially time and manpower, immediately eliminate most options.
- The fact that some of the goals are related means that making a decision about one of them closes down choices in others.
- Finally, the mix of staff skills and staff availabilities at the disposal of the project coordinator means that some alternatives are just not feasible.

By these means, the possible permutations of actions and resources reduce the ways in which a subproject's goals may be optimally achieved.

Staff with relevant expertise and experience were identified as a named link person to assume responsibility for each of the eight subprojects. These individuals were to become the knowledgeable operators who contributed to each subproject and liaised and collaborated with the IBL coordinator. Other staff with an interest in each area were co-opted. The IBL coordinator, working from a whole implementation perspective, ensured that the plan for the IBL implementation was not sub-optimized:

- making sure resources were distributed fairly between subprojects
- if there were inter-subproject dependencies, i.e. actions in one subproject that produce outputs needed by a second subproject, making sure that such events were synchronized.

In Step 4, the planned tasks and goals developed in earlier steps are documented as actions scheduled against the project calendar. A separate schedule, in the form of a Gantt chart, is shown for each of the eight subprojects in Figures 4.3 to 4.10. A brief overview of each schedule is given here – detailed discussions of the subprojects are given in Part III of this book.

Each of the eight subproject Gantt charts shows the overall goal of that component of the implementation project. The name of the subproject operator – the person with the main responsibility for achieving the subproject goal – is also shown. This individual is consulted by the IBL coordinator about the relevant actions listed at the left of the chart: how long each activity is likely to take; when it can start; when it must finish. The estimated times are plotted against the project calendar which runs across the top of the matrix.

Subproject 1 Staff development (see Figure 4.3). A commitment to the provision of ongoing staff development and support is essential for successful implementation of IBL. A variety of programmes aimed at meeting the educational and training needs of academic and practice staff were developed. The different needs of each group were determined by the role each plays in relation to the IBL implementation process. The programme provided opportunities for individuals to participate appropriately prior to any involvement in the curriculum implementation, giving them active preparation for their role in IBL. It was expected that academic and practice staff would participate in Stages 1 and 2 of the three-stage programme before undertaking the role of an IBL facilitator.

Subproject 2 Communication system (see Figure 4.4). Mechanisms were instituted to keep staff and students informed of programme plans and the progress of the implementation, in order to improve communication. Raising awareness of the curriculum and its implementation ensured that IBL was given a high profile and that all staff and students received the same information.

Subproject 3 Classroom compass (see Figure 4.5) is the whole range of classroom based activities, processes and structures. A learning environment conducive to the IBL philosophy was created that was inclusive and designed to advance the student's education.

Subproject 4 Practice experience (see Figure 4.6). Student practice experience is a major element in their educational preparation. Allocation of IBL students to appropriate care settings that will enable them to participate, to provide nursing care and to develop professional competencies is of primary concern.

Subproject 5 Documentation (see Figure 4.7). Provision of documents for curriculum implementation is likely to place a considerable strain on resources when information is still largely paper-based. It was imperative that this aspect was coordinated and reviewed in line with other subprojects. In this way, consistency and quality of the information related to the programme was maintained.

Subproject 6 Electronic resources (see Figure 4.8). While the value of IT systems for supporting students' learning is widely acknowledged, student expectations of

INQUIRY-BASED LEARNING IMPLEMENTATION PLAN

Subproject 1: STAFF DEVELOPMENT
Goal: prepare academic and practice staff for their new role

subproject operator:

Actions	1999									2000			
	APR	MAY	JUN	JUL	AUG	SEP	OCT	NOV	DEC	JAN	FEB	MAR	APR
Academic facilitators' teambuilding study day									■	■			
Facilitators' three-day workshops										■	■		
Subject/module team workshops				■	■	■	■	■	■	■	■	■	■
Academic staff curriculum update sessions			■	■		■	■	■	■	■		■	
Information Management and Technology workshop										■			
Practice staff awareness programme	■	■	■	■	■	■	■	■					
Practice supervisors' and mentors' preparation							■	■	■			■	■
Clinical practice supervisors' update sessions	■	■	■	■	■	■	■	■	■	■			
Academics and practice staff Away Day – launching the project					■								
Evaluate goals									■	■	■		

Figure 4.3 Gantt chart – Subproject 1: staff development (with examples of actions)

INQUIRY-BASED LEARNING IMPLEMENTATION PLAN

Subproject 2: COMMUNICATION SYSTEM
Goal: *improve communication with staff and students*

subproject operator:

Actions	1999									2000			
	APR	MAY	JUN	JUL	AUG	SEP	OCT	NOV	DEC	JAN	FEB	MAR	APR
Prepare directory of academics and practice staff									▓	▓			
Start academic facilitators' support group										▓	▓		
Prepare IBL notice board for students											▓	▓	
Project progress report to Curriculum Management Group									▓	▓	▓	▓	▓
Develop IBL information pack for practice areas							▓	▓	▓	▓	▓	▓	
Produce staff and student information handbooks							▓	▓	▓	▓	▓		
Obtain business cards and diary for academic facilitators								▓					
Present implementation plan to academic and practice staff	▓			▓		▓						▓	
Evaluate goals										▓	▓		

Figure 4.4 Gantt chart – Subproject 2: communication system (with examples of actions)

INQUIRY-BASED LEARNING IMPLEMENTATION PLAN

Subproject 3: CLASSROOM COMPASS
Goal: *create environment conducive to IBL philosophy*

subproject operator:

Actions	1999									2000			
	APR	MAY	JUN	JUL	AUG	SEP	OCT	NOV	DEC	JAN	FEB	MAR	APR
Identify field specific academic facilitators and module leaders		■	■	■									
Design activities timetable for academic facilitators					■	■							
Prepare student timetables						■	■	■	■	■			
Identify and prepare suitably sized rooms for IBL groups							■	■	■	■	■		
Prepare nursing skills laboratories							■	■	■	■			
Install science and skills laboratory equipment								■	■	■			
Design evaluation methods, tools and criteria								■	■	■			
Employ skills laboratory coordinator and technician							■	■					
Evaluate goal								■	■	■	■		

Figure 4.5 Gantt chart – Subproject 3: classroom compass (with examples of actions)

INQUIRY-BASED LEARNING IMPLEMENTATION PLAN

Subproject 4: PRACTICE EXPERIENCE
Goal: develop appropriate practice experience for students

subproject operator:

Actions	1999									2000			
	APR	MAY	JUN	JUL	AUG	SEP	OCT	NOV	DEC	JAN	FEB	MAR	APR
Identify practice areas for IBL student experience					▓	▓	▓						
Contribute to student placement allocation										░	░	░	
Develop practice staff handbook								▓	▓	▓			
Develop IBL practice supervisors register								░	░	░			
Arrange for provision of student nurse uniforms										▓	▓	▓	
Arrange for provision of work experience agreement										░	░	░	░
Evaluate goals									▓	▓	▓		

Figure 4.6 Gantt chart – Subproject 4: practice experience (with examples of actions)

INQUIRY-BASED LEARNING IMPLEMENTATION PLAN

Subproject 5: DOCUMENTATION
Goal: provide information related to the programme

subproject operator:

Actions	1999									2000			
	APR	MAY	JUN	JUL	AUG	SEP	OCT	NOV	DEC	JAN	FEB	MAR	APR
Develop learning packages													
Develop academic facilitators resource guide													
Develop students handbook													
Develop module assessment information: schedules, calendar, guidelines, assignments, criteria, etc.													
Develop module guides													
Develop practice assessment booklet													
Develop student portfolio document													
Evaluate goal													

Figure 4.7 Gantt chart – Subproject 5: documentation (with examples of actions)

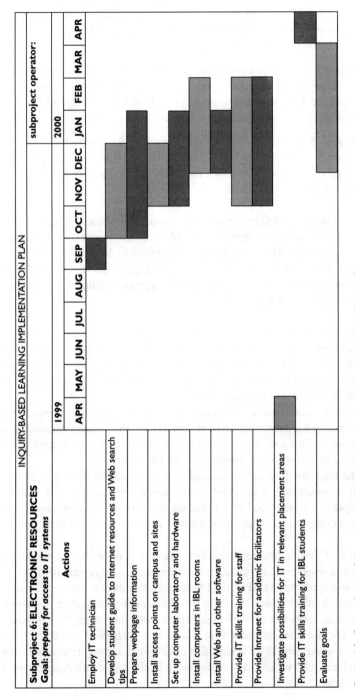

Figure 4.8 Gantt chart – Subproject 6: electronic resources (with examples of actions)

the type of information needed to advance their learning grows constantly so there is always a risk of under-provision. Virtually unlimited access has been provided to a variety of IT resources to benefit students and help them gain the knowledge and skills needed to enhance learning.

Subproject 7 Library resources (see Figure 4.9). IBL students can be expected to use the library more frequently and for longer periods than students following traditional teaching/learning approaches. Therefore the capability of existing resources and facilities requires reassessment to meet their needs.

Subproject 8 Media resources (see Figure 4.10). Operationalizing an IBL curriculum in which self-directed students require time-independent access to a wide range of information makes it necessary to provide a variety of audio-visual and other electronic equipment.

Obviously the scheduled activities shown for each subproject could be broken down further, and the project calendar could be given more precision by using weeks rather than months. There was a strong temptation to do just that initially – indeed a number of project management software packages were investigated by the IBL coordinator to see what a computer-assisted approach could offer. The notion was rapidly discarded for three reasons:

1　The philosophy and methodology of formal project management software packages appears to be irredeemably authoritarian and hierarchical. This is wholly incompatible with IBL concepts of self-directedness and facilitativeness – and seemed likely to cause considerable role confusion in staff who are both educators and on the project team.
2　A project management system running at a detailed level consumes a lot of data. Estimates from management and actuals from those doing the work have to be keyed in. This would put quite a heavy additional administrative burden on a resource that would be stretched to the limit anyway.
3　The high level model of the project represented by the Gantt charts of the eight subprojects was actually sufficient for the purposes of managing the implementation of the IBL curriculum. Project members could readily see what their contribution should be and how it fitted into the overall picture.

In Step 5 of the five planning steps (see Figure 4.2, page 38), the planned actions, designated resources and goals are communicated to everyone involved for validation and approval. At APU, the IBL coordinator gave a successful introductory presentation to the stakeholders on the Curriculum Management Group (CMG) – and subsequently to others involved in the curriculum – using the subproject Gantt charts. The documented plans were modified in the light of constructive criticism – always welcomed since it signifies conditional approval; after all, 'the more stakeholders who validate a plan, the more likely it is to be implemented' (Bruce and Langdon 2000: 37).

INQUIRY-BASED LEARNING IMPLEMENTATION PLAN

Subproject 7: LIBRARY RESOURCES
Goal: provide access to appropriate learning material

subproject operator:

Actions	1999									2000			
	APR	MAY	JUN	JUL	AUG	SEP	OCT	NOV	DEC	JAN	FEB	MAR	APR
Audit library in readiness to support IBL						■	■						
Locate appropriate learning material							■	■	■				
Set up workshops for student library skills development													■
Audit off-campus libraries								■					
Library staff awareness session										■			
Evaluate goal													■

Figure 4.9 Gantt chart – Subproject 7: library resources (with examples of actions)

Subproject 8: MEDIA RESOURCES
Goal: *provide quality support for media and equipment*

subproject operator:

Actions	1999									2000			
	APR	MAY	JUN	JUL	AUG	SEP	OCT	NOV	DEC	JAN	FEB	MAR	APR
Provide media resources in IBL rooms										■	■	■	
Provide reprographic materials					▒	▒	▒	▒	▒	▒	▒	▒	
Provide audiovisual aids in IBL rooms								■	■	■	■	■	
Arrange production of documents							▒	▒	▒				
Identify administrative staff to support IBL and IBL coordination						■							
Administrative staff awareness session							▒	▒	▒	▒	▒	▒	
Evaluate goals									■	■	■	■	

Figure 4.10 Gantt chart – Subproject 8: media resources (with examples of actions)

Contingency planning

There is no such thing as the perfect plan – where everything turns out just as we said it would – because our guesses about future events are based on the hope that what happened last time will happen next time, and that is not always so. But the future is not completely new, there is continuity with the past. We can expect some of our guesses to be right – if a supplier has always delivered on time in the past it is reasonable to expect that same good practice will be continued in future. With a new supplier we cannot be so certain and it is only prudent to entertain the possibility that the delivery may be late. A contingency plan specifies what we can do to reach our goals in spite of things going wrong. In the IBL implementation project, for example, contingency plans were made in case of:

- late delivery of equipment/material
- equipment failure
- staff lost to the project.

All of these problems occurred without adversely affecting the achievement of the project goals because their impact was offset by appropriate contingent actions. Late delivery, for instance, was offset by giving the procurement process more time – ordering early for an earlier delivery. Time contingencies are the most flexible and, more often than not, the least expensive option. If staff are lost to the project, the simplest contingency is to allow more time to complete tasks. If the lost staff is a specialist then the contingency might have to be bringing in a replacement. And if time itself is scarce – as it was in our case because of the heroic deadlines set for project completion – then additional staff have to be allocated so that tasks can be finished more quickly. Once appropriate contingencies have been specified, the arrangements have to be integrated into the project plan, as Bruce and Langdon (2000) advise, before it is presented to the CMG for ratification by stakeholders.

Finally, contingency planning only protects the project from expected problems. The unexpected is more difficult. We did build in a time contingency in the project plans for the supply of the special student chairs for the IBL rooms. It was generous enough to counter normal delay, but proved woefully inadequate when the chair factory caught fire.

Project implementation stage

Once the scheduled plans had been agreed by the CMG, implementation could begin to operationalize IBL philosophy and methodology in the pre-registration nursing programme. The mode of implementation of a whole integrated curriculum is analogous to launching a ship – everything has to be committed at the same time and it all has to work from day one. When the new students arrived in April 2000, they came into an IBL world – everywhere they went and everything they did was under the aegis of IBL.

There were problems of course – it is not possible to predict every eventuality. Live operation is bound to spring a few surprises; however, there were no major emergencies on this occasion. The success of the implementation was largely due no doubt to the quality and dedication of everyone involved. But it is also possible that the project planning and implementation benefited from the robust flexibility that is characteristic of self-directed thinking, feeling and doing.

Project evaluation stage

The IBL coordinator was accountable to the joint academic and service stakeholders for the success of the IBL implementation project and was therefore required to report the project's status at regular intervals. The achievement of the scheduled actions in each subproject was monitored. In reporting progress it was necessary to give an explanation for any slippage and indicate the steps that were being taken to recover and get back on schedule.

Conclusion

The IBL curriculum implementation project has been explored in this chapter in sufficient detail for others to model their own projects on what we have done at APU. What we have taken from the literature and found to be of value we are happy to pass on here. The most useful techniques were the simplest: breaking the project down into logical manageable subprojects; finding knowledgeable, motivated operators to champion each subproject; being realistic about what could go wrong and formulating appropriate contingency plans; using the sub-project schedules to monitor actions with the project team, and report progress to stakeholders.

Glossary of terms

Health authorities   These report to the Department of Health and are responsible for the strategic management of the primary and secondary care trusts that deliver healthcare at the local level.

National Health Service (NHS)   This was set up in the United Kingdom in 1948 to provide healthcare for all citizens based on need – not the ability to pay. Since it is funded by the taxpayer it is accountable to Parliament and managed overall by the Department of Health. It comprises a wide range of health professionals, support workers and organizations.

NHS trusts   These provide secondary care in the form of acute and specialized hospital and mental health services. Trusts attached to universities play a part in the education of health professionals.

Primary care trusts   These comprise general practitioners, nurses, health visitors, pharmacists and others delivering neighbourhood healthcare services.

Workforce Development Confederation (formerly known as NHS consortia) This organization brings together local NHS and private health-care employers to plan and develop the entire healthcare workforce. It reports to the Department of Health and is responsible for the education and training budget.

Chapter 5

Change management

Introduction

> Change is a process, not a destination. It never ends. Regardless of how successful you are this year, there is always next year.
>
> (Belasco 1992: 243)

It is good to be reminded that it is a changing world, that change is not an option, that it happens anyway, and it is continuous. What is an option is that we can induce a specific change of our own choosing: deciding when it starts, how it goes on and when it finishes – within the usual limits of success or failure that attend all human endeavours, that is. Changing things, like upgrading a computer for instance, is usually straightforward and requires minimal planning. Getting people to change is rarely or never straightforward. When the people are many and the change substantial, then a well-founded plan is mandatory. Implementing an integrated whole IBL curriculum into the pre-registration nursing programme certainly involved a lot of people. And the contemplated change was more than substantial, it was a paradigm shift that re-contoured the entire academic landscape and changed our world.

Staff reactions to change

How do I fit into this?

When the philosophy and methods of the incoming curriculum are, like IBL, very new and radically different, everyone has to review their role and responsibilities. Almost overnight, teacher-centred lecturing experience appears to lose its professional worth so that the lecturer with twelve years' know-how may feel they have little more to bring to the IBL staff development session than the lecturer with twelve months'. Viewed thus, effectiveness, self-esteem, perhaps even sense of identity count for little. The perception that the expert has been brought down to the level of a novice – by having to learn new ways of doing things – can provoke those who take it that way into a fight to preserve the pre-change differentials of power and status. Resistance may be a covert – or fully overt if there are enough resistors – attempt to derail the curriculum implementation.

Here we go again

With openness comes trust, with trust comes acceptance. If those initiating change do not present their rationale openly to those who are going to be affected, then the latter are bound to conclude it is not intended for their benefit. Feelings of mistrust and exclusion manifest themselves as fear and scorn towards the change initiators and stiffen resistance to any change proposed by them.

The managers do not know what they're doing

Staff really do have a different point of view from management. What seems like a benefit to one party, may look more like a disadvantage to the other – and vice versa. For example, increased productivity – a good thing from a management perspective – is not always seen as a benefit by those who actually have to set to and produce the extra output.

Management must demonstrate that they have taken the staff view into account – even when they are certain that the view is misconceived. The people affected by change initiated by others believe that their objections are well founded and they are sincere in that belief. And, for prudence's sake, the initiator of change should give some consideration to the possibility that they may be right.

Change model

> The key, of course, was to see that human change, whether at the individual or group level, was a profound psychological dynamic process that involved painful unlearning without loss of ego identity and difficult relearning as one cognitively attempted to restructure one's thoughts, perceptions, feelings, and attitudes.
>
> (Schein 2001: 1)

Schein is critiquing, in this quotation, Kurt Lewin's model of the human change process. The latter's work offers two insights that are of especial significance in the context of implementing self-directed learning. The first is to be reminded – in case we had overlooked the obvious – that human change can only come about as an outcome of learning. The second is that since change is a cognitive process, the use of any element of compulsion is likely to be ineffective and would certainly be inefficient. In accordance with IBL principles, change is best facilitated rather than forced. Human change is dependent upon the willing cooperation of staff in a three-step process of accepting the need for change, making the changes and actualizing

CHANGE STEPS	CHANGE ISSUES	DESIRED OUTCOMES	ACTIONS THAT FACILITATE CHANGE
1 Unfreezing existing beliefs	Existing beliefs must be changed before present attitudes can be changed	• Resistance to change is overcome, or seriously weakened • Existing beliefs are seen to be unsatisfactory • Determination to change	• Create open communications • Build confidence and trust • Promote staff participation • Keep staff up to date with relevant information • Cultivate good relationships
2 Changing	Change must be desired and recognized as necessary	• Readiness to change • Explore and try out new attitude, new behaviour	• Encourage active involvement in learning new attitude, behaviour • Establish two-way relationship • Provide guide/mentor for staff
3 Refreezing	Commit to permanent change	• Conviction that change will benefit self and group • Confident and self-assured about new attitude, new behaviour and new way of thinking	• Reinforce change with positive feedback from others • Reward the change appropriately

Figure 5.1 The change steps and action plan

the new belief, attitude and behaviour. This process is succinctly expressed in Lewin's powerful metaphor of unfreezing, changing and refreezing which provides us with the basis of a framework for planning change (see Figure 5.1).

Step 1: unfreezing The 'stability of human behaviour [is] based on "quasi-stationary equilibria"' (Schein 2001) – or, in more familiar language, a form of cognitive homeostasis in which one's inner conviction that what one believes is true balances out external arguments to the contrary. Unfreezing occurs when new information discredits the individual's belief, resistance crumbles, and the individual is left open to new learning experiences. However, individuals in this condition are also left wide open to self-doubt. If one could be so wrong about that, how much else of what one believes is also not true? If a core belief is threatened then self-doubt could trigger a descent into a sense of lost identity. The role of the initiator of change during this period of 'painful unlearning' is to provide psychological support – to be open, informative and involved. Left to flounder in anxiety and fear, the individual might retreat into a state of denial – stalling the unfreezing process and returning to the former belief.

Step 2: changing Change is more complete and enduring when the need for change is fully accepted and individuals want to learn. The change initiator facilitates the relearning process by encouraging staff to be actively involved in exploring and acquiring the new beliefs, attitudes and behaviour, by guiding them towards appropriate learning experiences as their mentor and role-model.

Step 3: refreezing Certainty that the new belief, attitude and behaviour are going to be advantageous to the individual, the rest of the staff and the health schools reinforces what has been learned. Objective evidence that confirms the worth of the change adds further reinforcement – in the IBL context that feedback would be student evaluation of the success of the tutorial process.

When staff have been instruments of their own change, through active learning, their confidence in the validity of the new view is soundly based. Cognitive homeostasis is re-established: one's conviction that one's belief is true balances out external contradictory arguments. This is refreezing – a state in which one continues until, at some future time, doubt sets in again. Refreezing is most likely to be successfully achieved when the new belief, attitude and behaviour is constructed from active learning, especially in a group.

Constructed knowledge is thoroughly integrated in the individual's existing knowledge base and is therefore entrenched and stable. Learning that comes from identifying with a role model may not be such a close fit with the personality of the individual. If the individual cannot fully identify psychologically and intellectually with the role model, the fit might be so poor that the new beliefs are not integrated and do not take. Refreezing may not take place, the new belief will be unlearned, and any change undone.

When individuals undergo change as a group they emerge from the process with group norms that support the new belief, attitude and behaviour. Refreezing is successful. But if a changed individual returns to a social environment which has norms that sustain the old beliefs the social pressure to conform is likely to prevent refreezing – and the change is not stabilized. Incidentally, this tendency to revert to the pre-change condition – under the influence of dominant cultural norms that are antagonistic to the new belief, attitude and behaviour – is a compelling argument for implementing a whole IBL curriculum.

Sources of resistance to change

Resistance can originate in individuals and groups, even the whole institution. The impulse to conservativism makes it hard for individuals and groups to give up familiar beliefs, attitudes and behaviours. Since 'individuals at every level in the organization are potentially liable to feel threatened by change' (Cole 1996: 193), change initiators should allow for a degree of resistance in their plans and have a strategy in place to deal with it. The change plan must be comprehensive enough to address change anxieties from a variety of sources. Examples of some encountered by the author at APU include:

- resentment of control
- insecurity
- social loss
- inconvenience.

Resentment of control

The things individuals do and use in the course of the daily routine soon become so familiar to them that they adopt them as being their own. When a large-scale change is proposed, they are shocked to discover how little really belongs to them – as educators, not even the tools of their trade – and therefore how little control they have over what is going to happen. Even the recognition that the change might be for the good did not necessarily outweigh the resentment felt by some that their normal method of delivering the programme had been made obsolete.

Insecurity

Doing the same things the same way for a long time creates a working environment and cultural ambience that is comfortable and, perhaps more significantly, comforting. To have the certainties of daily life removed – especially the simple undemanding customs and routines of a mainly teacher-centred programme – and replaced by the wholly different, advanced, active, personally demanding IBL approach – was undoubtedly unsettling and created feelings of insecurity in some colleagues.

Social loss

Change that affects the social environment can result in physical and psychological social loss. When an individual is physically lost to the group, because they have been given new responsibilities and join another group, the overall dynamic of the original group is diminished. But even if contact continues, new responsibilities generate a psychological distance that redefines the old relationship. The IBL implementation created a noticeable social upheaval when logistical constraints dictated a phased entry of lecturers into the staff development programme for IBL facilitators. The first group was made up of volunteers. Understandably, given the intensive IBL environment in which they found themselves, they rapidly formed into a tight-knit, motivated group. The new facilitators had new work patterns, new and different documentation, were involved in curriculum development activities and attended facilitator support group meetings. They were seen by those left behind in the 'old' programmes as a privileged elite. Awareness sessions and briefings could not bridge the gap between the two groups and there was a detectable loss of motivation and self-doubt in some staff.

Inconvenience

The introduction of the IBL philosophy and methodology into the pre-registration nursing programme generated massive change: new modules, new procedures, new techniques, new ways of thinking, feeling and doing. All this had to be learned by staff to a level of competence that would enable them to come in on implementation day and perform the duties of a full-time IBL facilitator with skill and confidence. The task of acquiring such a large amount of new information in a relatively short time was demanding, physically and mentally. Although many staff found this an entirely enjoyable experience, this extra workload was additional to the normal schedule of lecturing responsibilities. Everybody to a lesser or greater degree found it inconvenient. The negative impact of the start-up workload persisted for some time. It took approximately a year for many of the academic staff, and some practitioners, to finally accept that the IBL curriculum was viable, successful and here to stay.

Approaches to reducing resistance

Communication and education

Awareness sessions were held for academics and practitioners – the latter on location at Trust sites. Sessions were also provided in-house for other staff affected directly or indirectly by the changes, such as library and administrative staff. The main aims of the awareness sessions were:

- To keep staff fully informed about what was happening and what was proposed – demonstrating the openness of communications.
- To discuss the reasons for change: the shortcomings of the current approach, the benefits the new IBL approach will bring to those delivering and supporting the curriculum – personally, professionally and institutionally.
- To provide a platform for consultation: for staff to raise concerns, to make their objections known, to offer advice and suggestions – demonstrating that the views and feelings of staff are respected, valued and would be accommodated if possible and reasonable.
- To identify project team members available for follow-up queries and individual consultation.

The format of the awareness sessions was kept simple, flexible and informal. This was an unfreezing activity and we wanted staff to be as frank and open as possible with us. Together as a group we explored the areas and topics of interest and concern, such as:

- What needed to be changed, and why?
- Can it be changed?
- What cannot be changed?
- How do I have to change?
- Can I do it by myself?
- How do I get others involved?

All this is, of course, very reminiscent of what happens in a facilitated IBL group tutorial session, both in purpose and method – underlining the fact that change is a learning process.

Involvement and participation

Staff development – often with the assistance of external facilitators with relevant expertise – was the means by which all staff with a role in the delivery of the IBL curriculum became involved in the project. (The staff development programme for the IBL implementation is the subject of a later chapter.) Staff with additional responsibilities, such as module leaders, had further participation in curriculum development activities. The changing and refreezing steps which complete the change process take place during staff development.

Ongoing support

The mainstream programme for change was a satisfactory method of helping staff to move from the more teacher-centred to the new student-centred curriculum. Ongoing support was available for those who found acceptance and adjustment difficult – although time and patience were sometimes all that was required. Conversely, there were those whose enthusiasm outran their strength, or who had performed a particularly demanding task, who also needed appropriate support.

Conclusion

The scope and numbers involved in implementing an integrated whole IBL curriculum in a pre-registration nursing programme make it a very large project indeed. However, no matter how large the scale of a project might be, everything to do with change has to be carried out at the level of the individual – because human change depends upon the cognitive restructuring of individual thoughts, perceptions, feelings and attitudes. In our own efforts to manage change at APU, we designed, provided opportunities, and carried through an open-door, catch-all, supportive strategy for change that was intended to make sure that each of these individuals received the information, care and attention they needed to make a successful transition of the change process.

Part III

Operational practicalities

The subprojects

Chapter 6

Subproject 1:
staff development

Introduction

Making provision for the development of staff is an investment in the human capital of an enterprise. The sought after return on investment in this case was the successful implementation of an educationally advanced curriculum for pre-registration nursing programmes that promised positive academic and professional benefits over the short, medium and long terms. Naturally, where there is a 'high payoff potential . . . it is important to design and implement an effective [staff development] programme' (Hitchcock *et al.* 1993: 295).

There is a negative pressure that comes into play as well – stemming from the truism that 'the higher the profit, the higher the risk'. The cost of failure to achieve staff effectiveness in the delivery of the new curriculum would be proportionately high too. In the worst case scenario, a flawed attempt to implement IBL at the institutional level would have an adverse effect on academic results that threatens, in turn, recruitment, then funding and, sooner or later, the survival of the institution itself.

A similar profit and risk equation operates at the level of individual staff as well. The implementation of IBL brings into play new educational goals and strategies that call for new ways of thinking, feeling and doing. Anything less than a thorough root and branch remodelling of the staff development programmes for academics and practitioners is liable to leave staff anxious about their preparedness for their new roles (Doring *et al.* 1995). The cost of failure to design personal and professional development programmes that meet the needs of staff includes highly negative potential consequences on job satisfaction, career advancement and even employability.

In the event, the partnership of APU health schools and local Workforce Development Confederation regarded effective staff development of academics and practitioners as not just important but an inescapable prerequisite for the radical change from largely traditional methods of instruction to IBL, and made appropriate commitments of time and financial resources to this aspect of the project. Academics had to be prepared for a number of new educational roles – curriculum planners, IBL module leaders and facilitators. Practitioners needed to be prepared for their role in implementing IBL in the practice setting as mentors and supervisors for students. All this to allow implementation of the new curriculum in less than two years.

It has been observed that staff should not be expected to undertake the role of facilitator (and this is equally true for any other role that an academic or practitioner may perform in the IBL curriculum) 'without attending one or more staff development sessions' (David *et al*. 1999: 59). The need for physical attendance at sessions brings up two big obstacles faced by staff developers: staff availability and programme accessibility. From the outset, the APU health schools and Workforce Development Confederation understood that everyone concerned with the delivery of the pre-registration nursing programme should participate in suitable staff development – no matter how peripheral their involvement might be. Accordingly, the support of heads of division in the health schools and of practice managers in the trusts was sought to arrange for all staff to be available at some time for IBL staff development programme sessions. This is not simply a matter of reallocating resources so that staff can be released at appropriate times in appropriate numbers. Line managers had also to deal with the perennial problem of identifying and encouraging staff who are reluctant to change – either because they prefer to continue as they are, or because they are fearful of change itself.

The APU health schools adopted a staff development programme design strategy not dissimilar to that advocated by Hitchcock *et al*. (1993), namely:

- appoint an effective leader
- develop a specific strategy
- consult experts
- involve others in planning
- intervene to change the institutional environment
- establish a staff development evaluation programme.

This strategy was informed and refined with know-how gathered during visits to other universities and contributed to by experts on visits to APU, together with our own experience. The outcome of this process was a three-stage staff development programme for academics and nurse practitioners.

'A continuing programme of staff development is part of quality management' (David *et al*. 1999: 59). With this in mind, the programme was designed to be accessible, flexible and adaptive over time as new development needs evolve.

Staff views and beliefs about teaching and learning

'The path from lecturer to facilitator is often an uneasy one' (Little 1998: 121). To take an educator's beliefs from the traditional end of the teaching–learning spectrum and replace them with beliefs from the opposite end of that spectrum is notoriously problematic – especially if the original beliefs were implanted as a student teacher, more especially if they have been subsequently reinforced by years of successful and competent practice. Whatever relative position an educator might occupy on the teaching–learning continuum, the move to IBL modes of thinking and behaving will require a questioning of, and reflection upon, the philosophical rationale for long-held beliefs about how students learn and the role of the educator in that activity. Questioning and reflecting are of course key features of the IBL methodology so, paradoxically, in self-examination of their current beliefs traditional educators find themselves, willy-nilly, already beginning to use the tools of IBL. This early initiation might to some degree help to smooth the path from lecturer to facilitator, easing the anxieties of transition from old ways of thinking to new.

But 'if the required changes are perceived to be too great or too fast in relation to their existing interpretational schema' (Creedy *et al*. 1992: 729) then lecturers will be less willing to modify their beliefs. One such great change in IBL is the redistribution of educational authority and responsibility. The paradigmatic shift from teacher-centredness to student-centredness obsoletes much of the educator's existing repertoire of traditional pedagogic skills. Techniques acquired with no small effort, honed perhaps through a long professional life until they have become second nature, are relegated to the back of the cupboard – to be taken out only on those relatively few occasions when a lecture is judged to be the method of choice.

It is understandable, then, if lecturers are sometimes reluctant to change when the adoption of new beliefs means discarding hard won expertise. Clearly what any staff development programme must do before it does anything else is show participants how the new beliefs 'offer more to educators than the conceptions they currently hold' (Creedy *et al*. 1992: 732).

Role change

Because there appear to be many superficial physical correspondences in the functions of facilitating and lecturing – an academic, some students, a room with tables and chairs, whiteboard, flipcharts and so on – the realization that there is, on closer acquaintance, little common ground between them comes as an early shock to most participants in staff development. Pedagogic skills do not exist in a value-free conceptual vacuum – they are the physical expression of an underlying philosophy. Lecturing and facilitating are completely different because the former is a physical expression of teacher-centredness and the latter of student-centredness.

Whenever a particular technique is used, the philosophy that informs that technique comes alive and manifests itself in the classroom. A demonstration perhaps of Marshall McLuhan's dictum about the medium being the message (cited by Ebersole 1995). So, to lecture effectively, the educator is obliged to be dominant. In so doing, authoritarianism is made concrete and beliefs and attitudes that are antagonistic to IBL steal back into the classroom and derail the IBL tutorial process. The change of role from lecturer to facilitator 'demand[s] a relinquishing of the usual power relationships which occur between educator and students' (Van Niekerk and Van Aswegen 1993: 38). The relinquishment of those authoritarian power structures must be accompanied by the abandonment of all the techniques that depend upon teacher-dominance, to prevent the later re-emergence of concepts antithetical to IBL.

A second shock: what the lecturer knows already about their own area of specialist expertise will be of limited value when they take on the role of IBL facilitator. Subject knowledge – so important to lecturing – may be a hindrance to facilitation. In IBL, educators 'become facilitators of learning, guiding the students by appropriate questions' (Walton and Matthews 1989: 551). Crucially, the facilitators' questions are not concerned with content but with how the students are setting about the business of learning. In effect, if the exploration of the domain is carried out effectively then the requisite knowledge will be found – that is, learned – by the students.

If the educator is a subject expert, however, they face a dilemma – do they lecture or do they facilitate? Being expert in the subject may encourage them to contribute to the group's discussion of content, necessarily entering into the learning process from whence it is not possible for them to simultaneously facilitate that process (Philips and Philips 1993). The educator might ask such loaded questions that the group is steered straight to what the students need to know – need to know as defined by the educator, of course, so in reality the outcome is the same as might have been reached in a lecture. In this way, possession of subject expertise can interfere with the tutorial process and deny students some of the benefit of IBL. Unsurprising then, that De Grave *et al.* (1999) found that students rated facilitators whose style of facilitation focused on the learning process as more effective than those whose style focused on content.

There is a third shock awaiting the educator changing roles from lecturer to facilitator. The sense of gratification and self-worth that some lecturers might get – by being the source of all wisdom and its principal conduit – are forever lost with the change of title. In a student-centred curriculum, the students soon become accomplished at self-directed learning. It follows, by reason of symmetry, that if the students are largely self-directed, then the educator's role is secondary in the learning process. Researchers have already found that students on a PBL programme 'function independently of the facilitator at least 90 per cent of the time' (Zeitz and Paul 1993: 203). The contribution that the facilitator makes to student learning is not overt and, even when done well, may not be acknowledged as a contribution by the students who directly benefit from it. The facilitator works in the margins – a collaborator and helper whose greatest achievements will be enjoyed by others. Good reasons for the staff developer to ensure that the programme design recognizes that 'lecturer preparation and continued support is vital to change pedagogical attitudes and overcome lecturer discomfort' (Haith-Cooper 2000: 270).

Planning staff development

The indispensable need for staff development has been continually emphasized in the literature. 'Extensive and well attended faculty development workshops for tutors are imperative' (Walton and Matthews 1989: 552) – an admonition repeated by Creedy and Hand (1994) and Alavi (1995).

In 1998 APU began work on the design and development of the new IBL curriculum for pre-registration nursing – due for implementation in April 2000 with a first intake of 148 Diploma in Higher Education (Nursing) students. A staff development programme was scheduled to begin at the same time, to run in parallel with the curriculum development project. In recognition of its pivotal role in the successful implementation and subsequent operation of the new curriculum, the staff development programme was well supported by the Curriculum Steering Group – which comprised senior Workforce Development Confederation personnel and senior academic managers.

Staff development coordination

Hitchcock *et al.* (1993) make the simple point that a successful staff development programme is one that staff know about and want to attend. To give it the necessary high profile and credence, they suggest it should be coordinated by a senior manager experienced in staff development – with the resources to drive and direct the programme. An IBL coordinator meeting these requirements was appointed and given responsibility for implementing the operational elements of the curriculum – a remit that included the preparation of the IBL facilitators, practitioners and others involved in the delivery of the new curriculum, for their various roles. This appointment was made about fifteen months prior to implementation – at least a year for the preparation of IBL facilitators in the run-up to the start date of the new curriculum is recommended by Murray and Savin-Baden (2000).

The role of the IBL coordinator in staff development includes:

- developing programmes
- ensuring delivery of the agreed programme as scheduled
- supporting and motivating the staff responsible for delivering sessions
- communicating updates/changes to staff
- delivering sessions
- quality assuring sessions by evaluation and feedback.

Types of staff development strategies

A range of approaches has been implemented and evaluated at APU. The most widely used strategies are:

- Short programmes, for example, workshops and seminars: workshops especially have proved to be the most effective and this, together with their short duration, has made them the preferred, and most frequently used, method of developing academic and practice staff.

- Courses: a planned postgraduate educational programme is offered as part of staff development at APU for those undertaking advanced studies – such as a Masters in Education. The course of study includes other modules of learning, but the principal focus for staff preparing for the role of facilitator is the masters level module 'Facilitating IBL'.
- Peer support group: planned occasions where facilitators meet to relate experiences and discuss problems, to share ideas and offer solutions.

Developing a staff development strategy

The IBL coordinator at APU agreed a strategy with the Curriculum Steering Group for academic and practice staff development that matched the needs of staff, the health schools and the trusts. A variety of programmes were designed to address the different needs of the different roles: of academics – as IBL facilitators and module leaders – and of practice staff – as supervisors and mentors.

Staff development strategy for academics

In the run-up to implementation, academics from other institutions, expert in IBL or student-centred learning gave presentations and seminars at health schools level on the IBL tutorial method, the role of the facilitator, creating scenarios and structuring modules. Arrangements were made for the Curriculum Steering Group, the Curriculum Development Group, and other academic staff and practitioners, to visit Southampton University – who were already implementing enquiry-based learning in their pre-registration nursing programme. These information gathering exercises provided valuable insights into staff development and curriculum implementation that APU's planners and developers were able to draw upon in devising their own programmes. An early product of these investigations was the academic staff development strategy – delivered as a three-stage programme (see Figure 6.1).

Stage 1: developing awareness

Stage 1 is an awareness session that was started more than a year before implementation as a rolling programme to ensure that all academic staff had the opportunity to attend a range of study days and workshops. Outside experts on PBL/EBL student-centred learning were brought in from other universities to lead these sessions. Initially this was done simply to avoid reinventing the wheel, but the practice has been retained because it maximizes the impact of new concepts and attitudes on the participants – leaving a lasting first impression of the power and range of IBL philosophy and methodology. APU academics who had observed and participated in sessions provided by the external experts facilitated awareness sessions for colleagues who had been unable to attend.

STAGE	AIMS	STRATEGY
1 Developing awareness	• To begin the cultural change • To understand IBL, its philosophy and its process	• A series of workshops and study days delivered for all academic staff on raising awareness and introducing IBL as a model for curricular development. These sessions are led by guest speakers/experts in the area of IBL • A series of workshops on writing scenarios
2 Preparation of staff for their role as IBL facilitators	• To develop in-depth knowledge and skills to promote a culture that supports learning and growth	• Series of update sessions, delivered for all academic staff, on creating a picture of the students' experience and the operational aspects of IBL • Module leaders workshops for writing modules • Three-day workshop delivered for academics to prepare for their role as IBL facilitators. These sessions are led by internal and external facilitators. • Workshops to introduce IBL facilitators to the semester modules • 'Facilitating IBL' (30 credits) postgraduate module delivered for facilitators involved with the implementation of IBL/PBL curricula • Workshops for potential facilitators on understanding group dynamics, questioning skills, the collaborative process and Socratic dialogue. The sessions are led by cognitive behaviour therapists and other subject experts
3 Ongoing development and support	• To enhance facilitation in the context of IBL	• The three-day workshop continues – run once a year to prepare potential facilitators • Facilitators Peer Group meetings • Series of workshops/seminars as refresher programme and to update staff

Figure 6.1 Summary of three-stage academic staff development programme

Two-day workshops introduce academics to IBL so that they can begin to understand IBL theory and practice. Further two-day workshops focus on the writing of scenarios and the tutorial process.

Stage 2: preparation of staff for their role as IBL facilitators

On completing Stage 2, it is intended that attendees should have 'skill at facilitation and willingness to empower the students with the excitement of learning' (Woods 1994: 177). If these outcomes are not achieved – and subsequently, in their practice, facilitators are neither pedagogically adept nor capable of enthusing learners – then the educational consequences can be grave. An incompetent facilitator will not have the skills to initiate and sustain the tutorial process on which IBL depends. If the students involved are experienced and motivated enough to carry on without the help and guidance of a facilitator then that might limit the immediate damage. However, if the students are not educationally autonomic IBL veterans then what should have been an IBL session is likely to collapse, degenerating instead into some sort of teacher-directed model in which students are presented with subject content but never discover for themselves how to learn or be self-directed. It seems the incompetent facilitator is not as uncommon a figure as one would wish. Barrows (1986) identifies quality of facilitation as a widespread concern for schools using PBL.

In the traditional teaching model, lecturers gain and hold their posts in educational institutions by virtue of their understanding of some domain of knowledge. In IBL, subject expertise is, strictly speaking, irrelevant. Indeed, to the extreme IBL purist, content knowledge can be considered a liability in the educational process. The urge to share what one knows with others is all too human – for some of us, it must be said, is almost a compulsion. The downside of this otherwise innocent impulse is that it might tempt the educator into sounding forth on their specialist subject – instead of encouraging students to explore the topic for themselves.

This restriction is to be taken as a warning against giving out content knowledge with such unasked-for liberality that it actually undermines the IBL tutorial process. It is not intended as a perverse advocacy of ignorance as an educational resource. Just because being an expert facilitator is of more value than being a subject expert, as Barrows (1988) stressed, it does not follow that knowing nothing of the subject is wholly advantageous. As Davis *et al.* (1992) suggested, and Nayer (1995) later made emphatic, facilitators do, after all, have need of some understanding of the content of an IBL module and its scenario (a view endorsed by the author of this book). Some subject knowledge will help them to recognize the point at which group discussion becomes sterile, or when the group needs to change learning strategies because it is missing an important concept or overvaluing an insignificant one. APU develops existing staff with workshops that introduce IBL facilitators to the content of the semester's modules.

Three-day facilitators' workshop

> Teachers talk about teachings. Real teachers study their pupils as well. Most
> of all, teachers should be studied.
>
> (Musa Kazim, cited by Shah 1990: 241)

Figure 6.2 outlines the daily programmes of the three-day facilitators' workshop.
These have been held twice a year since January 2000 to motivate and enthuse
participants. The aim is to prepare staff, building up their confidence and capability
before they launch themselves into their new roles as IBL facilitators. The workshops are mandatory for all potential facilitators and are attended as an essential
adjunct to the induction process by all new academic staff. To date, the number
of participants at each workshop has ranged between twelve and twenty-two and
included staff from the four nursing fields – adult nursing studies, childhood studies,
mental health studies and learning disabilities studies – as well as social work
academics from APU, practice student facilitators from hospital trusts and, recently,

---

**INQUIRY-BASED LEARNING FACILITATORS'
WORKSHOP PROGRAMME**

Aim: To prepare academic staff for the role of facilitator

DAY 1
Registration and refreshments
Welcome and overview of the workshop and outcomes
Overview of the pre-registration nursing programme
Break
Facilitated IBL group work – STEP 1: EXPLORATION TUTORIAL
Lunch
Parallel resource sessions × 3[1]

- Using Library resources
- Assessment of theory and practice
- Roles and responsibilities in the Practice setting

Fixed-resource session – The role of the facilitator in enhancing learning[1]
Break
Parallel resource sessions × 3

- Clinical nursing skills
- Information management and technology/WebCT
- Practice placements

Non-facilitated IBL group work
Self-directed study (access resources/computer room)
Dinner

Figure 6.2 IBL facilitators' workshop programme outline

DAY 2
Breakfast
Fixed-resource session – The IBL tutorial process at APU
Break
Fixed-resource session – Questioning skills, giving and receiving feedback
Self-directed study (access resources/computer room)
Lunch
Fixed-resource session – Group dynamics
Break
Facilitated IBL group work – STEP 2: REVIEW TUTORIAL
Self-directed study (access resources/computer room)
Dinner
Opportunity to access resources

DAY 3
Breakfast
Fixed-resource session – Evaluation process and methods
Break
Facilitated IBL group work – STEP 3: CONSOLIDATION AND PLENARY
TUTORIALS
Lunch
Student portfolio
The role of the student facilitator
Non-facilitated IBL group work – Facilitators' action planning
Break
Plenary session – Sharing experiences
Close

Note I See page 89 for more details on parallel and fixed-resource sessions.

Figure 6.2 continued

a welcome attendee from another university. In a demonstration of a paradox often observed when real learning is taking place, the atmosphere is very relaxed but at the same time everyone is working very hard.

APU's off-campus conference centre, with its extensive training and residential facilities, was the venue of choice for the three-day workshops. The tranquillity of its rural setting and the well-appointed comfort of its full conference, small group and domestic facilities come together to meet the needs of both the outer and inner person. Daily cares can be cast off and, for a while, participants can immerse themselves in the rigours and rewards of scholarly activities in the company of their colleagues and peers.

The residential workshop provides the intellectual and psychological space, the motivation and material necessary for the successful transformation of participants from lecturer to facilitator in a number of ways. First, taking participants away from the responsibilities of the workplace and the home, unplugging them from their normal channels of communication, gives them the boon of uninterrupted time in which to study, reflect and learn. Second, bringing people together for a common purpose means that the common purpose becomes the main talking point. In this context, IBL topics dominate the social agenda – informal as well as formal – simply because that is the purpose for which everyone has come together. Third, there are opportunities for the private revelation of doubts and uncertainties to sympathetic and supportive peers – fears which may seem too slight or too foolish to express publicly in a formal setting but which, unattended to, may grow from neglect. Fourth, there are opportunities to share insights with other interested parties, and the time to explore and develop those understandings without intrusions or interruptions from the outside world.

There are substantial direct and indirect costs associated with the provision of a residential programme – institutional and individual, financial and personal. Given that the quality of the IBL curriculum is largely determined by the quality of the IBL facilitators – and that an intensive, focused programme is likely to be more efficient and more effective and have a reduced risk of failure than a more drawn out, fragmented, approach – the on-cost can be justified. This is not to say that, because of the greater educational and monetary benefits that ensue, residency should be made compulsory – there is a myriad of personal and familial obligations that might forbid such a draconian measure. The main objection is that compelling someone to learn in a certain way because that way suits the institution is not compatible with IBL's ruling principle of student autonomy.

The format of the three-day facilitators' workshop allows sufficient time for a deep, intense encounter with the IBL tutorial process which more authentically reproduces the IBL facilitator and student experiences.

The three-day workshop is organized and led by the IBL coordinator. It affords a thorough introduction to the educational philosophy of IBL and its methodology – showing how concepts, such as student-centredness, and core techniques, such as small-group work, are implemented and practised in the pre-registration nursing curriculum. The workshop addresses other relevant topics such as assessments, practice experiences, and the role of information technology.

For their simulated student experience, participants are split into small groups of ten to twelve members. Each group becomes an IBL tutorial group – with an expert facilitator provided as model and guide. The group chooses one of its number for the role of chair and another to be scribe. The group explores a relevant, realistic, but non-nursing, scenario. Throughout the three days of the workshop the participants also have opportunities to try out facilitation for themselves and to observe colleagues practising their facilitator skills. This approach is recommended for potential facilitators by Wilkerson and Hundert (1998) – the educational power and learning intensity of IBL accurately reproduced for, and actively experienced by, those in the staff development programme as if they, themselves, were IBL students.

A resource room in the conference centre is set up with all the documentation for the pre-registration nursing programme, the IBL tutorial process and the facilitators' role, with other related material for the general enlargement of participants' knowledge bases. There are also copies of the 'Facilitator's Handbook' – developed by the author – which has proved to be a useful guide that takes in the background to IBL facilitation.

One-hour resource sessions are distributed throughout the three-day workshop to focus on lines of enquiry set off by the scenario. In the initial phase of staff development, some sessions were led by external consultants expert in student-centred learning. The involvement of external experts, especially at start-up of a new curriculum, increases the confidence in, and credibility of, the implementation project.

Since the three-day IBL workshop is, in itself, a practical demonstration of IBL in action, it concludes with participants reflecting on what they have learned and how – what had assisted or hindered the learning process for them. At the plenary session, they share those experiences and present their action plans – an empowering moment which acknowledges that a great leap forward has been made and commits participants to a future of continual professional and personal development.

The three-day workshops are formally evaluated using a Likert-type scale questionnaire to elicit participant satisfaction information. The evaluations of the six workshops offered between January 2000 and January 2002 by potential facilitators, other academics and those with complementary roles to the IBL nursing programme, have been very positive – a majority of participants reporting themselves satisfied, with better understanding of IBL, their roles and their responsibilities.

Postgraduate module in 'Facilitating Inquiry-Based Learning'

A postgraduate module, 'Facilitating Inquiry-Based Learning' (designed by the author and implemented in January 2002), is an optional element of the Masters Degree in Teaching and Learning at APU. Its aims are to help potential facilitators to prepare for their new roles, and to contribute to the advanced professional development of academic staff who are already experienced IBL facilitators. The module extends knowledge and deepens understanding of the theoretical dimensions of IBL. Consequently, it provides an even more compelling intellectual rationale for moving away from traditional teaching to student-centred and student-directed learning in general and IBL in particular. The new comprehensions gained are intended to enhance the range and power of facilitative skills to improve the effectiveness and subtlety of their use by academics in the IBL tutorial process.

The module is delivered once a year in a single semester over an elapsed duration of six months – a programme construction that leaves participants free to perform their day to day staff work activities. The module (see Figure 6.3) was first delivered to five academics – a mixed selection of external and APU staff contributing between them a diversity of experience, academic disciplines and subject areas. The flexibility and adaptability inherent in an IBL oriented programme easily accommodate such a variety of input – the IBL process itself being fuelled, of course, by the range of differences in prior knowledge and perspective.

1   An Induction Day is held a month prior to the commencement of the programme. Participants are introduced to the module and an opportunity provided for them to begin to develop collaborative relationships with each other and with their facilitator.

2   This stage is delivered over a three-day period (optionally residential). The practical sessions include the use of the IBL tutorial process in a way that reproduces the experience of IBL students.
    (See Appendix 1, page 138, one student's reflections on the residential workshop.)

3   Participants are required to undertake a virtual IBL group exercise (based on a storyboard approach) during self-directed learning time. They are encouraged to work from the module Web pages. There is also a workbook (see Appendix 2, page 139, for an example exercise). The module uses a virtual IBL student group to stimulate and challenge participants to build skills and knowledge about working with small groups of students.

4   There are three additional study days in the semester for shared learning and peer support.

Figure 6.3 An outline of the postgraduate module programme 'Facilitating Inquiry-Based Learning'

Introduction to semester modules

At one-day workshops, facilitators who are not expert in the topics they will be involved with meet the module leaders responsible for the subject in the coming semester. These workshops are scheduled to occur about six weeks before the start of the module. The facilitators receive a pack of advance copies of the Facilitator's Module Guide and the module timetable for familiarization before attending the workshop. At the workshop, the module scenarios, learning outcomes, assessment requirements, module guidelines and resource sessions are appraised and discussed. Other non-academic matters are also dealt with, such as module administration, placements allocation, attendance requirements and registration, and IBL room arrangements. The one-day workshops are acknowledged to be essential by staff and are invariably well-attended. Questions can be asked, misunderstandings brought out and corrected, and any anxieties about readiness or competence addressed and allayed.

Stage 3: ongoing development and support

The overall purpose of this stage of the academic staff development programme (see Figure 6.1, page 67) is to enhance facilitation in the context of IBL. There are four main reasons for development. First, the acquisition of any domain of knowledge proceeds incrementally – IBL is no exception. There are regular sessions which progressively broaden and deepen understanding and enlarge and refine the repertoire of methods. Second, at the end of each module and each semester,

Staff development topics	Event facilitator
• The art of skilful questioning	External consultant
• Managing and facilitating small groups	External consultant
• Revisiting the IBL tutorial process	In-house
• Using reflective frameworks	In-house
• Managing conflict within the group	External consultant
• Information management and technology in the IBL programme	In-house
• Using WebCT	In-house
• Facilitators' semester fair	Internal and external contributors

Figure 6.4 Examples of ongoing staff development events organized at APU

facilitators complete evaluation questionnaires. In these, facilitators identify those areas of their practice that they believe would benefit from further development. Third, staff need to be updated on curriculum developments. Fourth, enthusing others can be exhausting, so facilitators may need to be refreshed and revitalized. Some examples of ongoing staff development for IBL facilitators are shown in Figure 6.4.

Facilitator peer group meetings

IBL facilitator peer group meetings are a regular forum for debate on the IBL philosophy and facilitation methodology, and any current IBL curriculum implementation issues. Sharing ideas about, and experiences of, IBL facilitating is, in effect, self-directed staff development. The general aim of the get-togethers was that participants should benefit, professionally and personally, from the opportunity to air concerns and get expert and sympathetic advice from their peers – in short, all the advantages of collegial support.

In the first two years of IBL implementation, the first-year student cohort facilitators met once a week, and the second and third year student cohort facilitators once a fortnight for two hours. New facilitators joined the weekly meeting. During the second year attendance at the meetings declined sharply – with, typically, only about 50 per cent of facilitators turning up. The main cause of falling numbers was competition from other work commitments. A second, more worrying, possibility was that perhaps some facilitators had relapsed to their former traditional teaching beliefs – or perhaps had never fully relinquished them. Such facilitators may have become disaffected – possibly by the stress of the daily conflict between what they wanted to do and what was expected of them.

To address these matters, a 'semester fair' has been organized – to be held twice a year beginning in September 2002 – for all staff involved in the implementation of the IBL curriculum, particularly facilitators. The purpose of the fair is to get reacquainted with core concepts of IBL, to revisit the facilitator's role, and get an update on the current status of modules and practice placements. There are drop-in stalls for all the major curriculum related concerns and issues, for example:

- programme modules
- clinical skills laboratory
- practice placements
- library resources
- information management and technology
- assessment
- evaluation
- the IBL tutorial process.

When the IBL curriculum had been implemented for a full year, a Celebration Day was held to give thanks for the success of the project, review the role of the facilitator, and to pay tribute to our facilitators' achievements. A special guest facilitator on this happy occasion was Dr Christine Alavi, the noted PBL proponent.

Staff development strategy for practitioners

The role of the academic in the pre-registration nursing programme is radically transformed – from lecturer to facilitator – with the implementation of an IBL curriculum. Practice supervisors – experienced nurse practitioners who have completed an approved teaching and assessing in clinical practice programme – must undergo a similar radical transformation in attitudes and behaviour to meet the learning needs of IBL student nurses in the practice setting. If nurse practitioners are not prepared educationally to a sufficient degree then the methods they employ to facilitate student learning are likely to be inadequate – as seen by White *et al.* (1993).

Practice supervisors are key to linking theory to practice, partly by creating appropriate learning situations and opportunities but also, importantly, by virtue of being potent nursing role models. Unsurprisingly, in a vocational profession, nursing students seem far more prone to model their behaviour on practitioners than on academics. Thus practice supervisors have a special responsibility to ensure that their behaviour as supervisors of student learning is reinforced by – rather than contradicted by – their behaviour as practitioners. The collaborative links that already existed were strengthened to draw practitioners and academics closer together into a single culture of shared beliefs and approaches. The responsibility for spreading the IBL philosophy and delivering practice staff development was assigned to the nursing field leaders and committed academic colleagues with expertise and experience of the IBL curriculum. By keeping the lines of communication short and clear in this way it was hoped to avoid the drift-off message that can occur when delivery is too decentralized.

In collaboration with the IBL coordinator, APU's academic nursing educators and curriculum planners had to design and implement a staff development strategy for practitioners that, first, ensured that the delivery of the IBL curriculum is seamless – wherever learning takes place and whoever guides and supports that learning – and, second, that the student experience in the practice setting is not contaminated by professional attitudes and conduct that are incompatible or antagonistic to IBL.

STAGE	AIMS	STRATEGY
1 Developing awareness	• To understand IBL, its philosophy and its process	• Road shows delivered between January 1999 and November 1999 at Hospital Trust sites • Trust representatives request sessions in liaison with IBL coordinator
2 Preparation of staff for their role as IBL practice supervisors	• To develop in-depth knowledge and skills to promote a culture that supports learning and growth	• Half-day workshop delivered to practice supervisors in core and associate placements on 'the operational aspects of IBL in practice settings'
3 Ongoing development and support	• To enhance practice supervision/facilitation in the context of IBL	• Half-day workshop run once in each semester to prepare potential supervisors and to inform other staff whose roles complement the IBL process • Informal IBL and curriculum update delivered by link academics to staff in their practice areas • Practice supervisors update session on IBL to develop awareness – includes the operational aspects of IBL in practice settings • Helpline: Academic Facilitator Contact Directory provided for staff in all placement areas • IBL information packs sited in all practice placement areas where students are allocated

Figure 6.5 Summary of the staff development programme for practitioners

There is little published material on what practice supervisors should be doing to support the IBL curriculum, and less on how best to prepare them for the changes in their role. Accordingly, APU developed its three-stage programme for practitioner staff development from first principles (see Figure 6.5).

Stage 1: developing awareness

Road shows were delivered to practice staff at the Hospital Trust sites on the students' practice placement circuit. The aim was to give practitioners an understanding of IBL's philosophy, its methodology, the new demands it would make on practice supervision and the impact on the ward environment.

Stage 2: preparation of staff for their role as IBL practice supervisors

Half-day workshops go more deeply into the operational implications of IBL and the changes to practice supervision methodology. Responsibility for continuity and consistency of application of the student-centred, facilitative, approach to learning passes from the academic facilitator to the practice supervisor when students go on placement. The practice supervisors gain an understanding of IBL, of its methodology and of facilitation, so that they are competent to implement IBL in the practice setting.

Stage 3: ongoing development and support

In the first two years following implementation of the IBL curriculum, a half-day workshop was held once in each semester to prepare potential practice supervisors and to inform other staff with roles that complement the IBL process. There is a variety of ongoing support. Academic facilitators are assigned to a practice link area where they join with practice supervisors in informal IBL and curriculum update sessions. There are more structured update sessions to refresh and extend practice supervisors' understanding of IBL and its operational application. The effectiveness of practice staff development is evaluated – in the main feedback has been positive.

Conclusion

A range of staff development programmes has been designed and delivered to prepare and sustain academic and practice staff involved in pre-registration nursing education in their roles in delivering the IBL curriculum. The success of the IBL implementation means that the pressure on the staff development programme to prepare new facilitators, to further enhance the knowledge and skills of experienced facilitators, and to prepare and support practice supervisors proceeds apace. Professional enthusiasm has been such that APU now offers a postgraduate module in 'Facilitating IBL' to meet the higher aspirations of academic staff.

The staff development programme has been shown to strengthen relationships within the academic community and with practitioners. Perhaps because facilitating concentrates so much attention on the learning process, a number of innovative proposals to improve operational effectiveness have been put forward for implementation. Like IBL itself, the staff development programme is a group activity, a shared endeavour that has generated an intellectual and psychosocial environment that is tuned to the philosophy and conducive to the practice of IBL.

Chapter 7

Subproject 2: communication system

Introduction

From the outset it was recognized that the quality of communication was going to be crucial to the successful implementation of IBL. Unless the philosophy and methodology of IBL was shared and understood by a very large majority of those involved in the new curriculum, there would be an imperfect acceptance of change and a consequent risk that the implementation would fail. The Curriculum Management Group was also mindful that the project should be given a high profile to generate the intensity of interest and enthusiasm needed to get things moving and maintain momentum. Even with high levels of motivation and acceptance, successful implementation still needs effective project management and that too is dependent upon the flow of accurate, timely information. It was for these reasons that the communication system was made a subproject in its own right and started early in the planning stage.

The core process that defines communication is 'the giving and receiving of information' (Andrews 1995: 56). Only when information is shared can it be said that communication has taken place. The information giver cannot be sure that something has been shared unless there is feedback to that effect from the receiver. The feedback may reveal that the information has not after all been received – it was misinterpreted, or, the significant information went unseen, buried in superfluous data, or was made unintelligible by an immoderate use of jargon.

Expressing information in terms that are clear and unambiguous is difficult enough. Limiting what is communicated to just the information that the giver wants to share, is well-nigh impossible. No matter how considered the content, the tone, language, presentation, medium and means of distribution, some extra information is always conveyed unintentionally. Humans are adept at going beyond what is stated to what is implied, deducing what has not been mentioned, assessing the degree of spin. Every deliberate communication between humans arrives at its destination tagged with a multitude of these unintentional micro-social, micro-political revelations. It is good sense, therefore, as well as good ethics, to be as open, honest and straightforward in one's communications with others as possible – leaving nothing discreditable to be read between the lines.

The first step was a survey of the current communications system in the APU health schools to identify which components would be of general use during the IBL implementation and to determine the gaps where new channels for the flow of project-specific information would need to be set up. It was obvious that the design of the communication channels should be in tune as far as practicable with IBL philosophy by being direct, two-way, flexible and non-authoritarian. The ideal format is that of the forum where the givers and receivers of information – whether students, practitioners or academics – can engage in a face-to-face dialogue where questions can be asked and answered, and concerns raised and addressed.

The main opportunities for the oral exchange of information are in team briefings, consultative committees, staff development workshops, and meetings of all sorts. Two of the reasons that 'no communication technique however technically advanced or sophisticated, improves upon face to face communication' (Andrews 1995: 63) are that it cycles so rapidly and it leaves no permanent record. In the verbal to and fro, communications can be reinforced and clarified, corrected or refuted, quickly and with the minimum of drama.

The second consideration was taking pains to ensure that information should be presented as clearly and relevantly as possible. This could be achieved with greater certainty if communications recognized and took into account the local circumstances of recipients. A third consideration was the timing of the initial announcement – which would of necessity immediately reveal the radical nature of the projected changes. It was felt that an announcement of major change that lacked requisite specifics about how it would impact individuals would be bound to produce a climate of anxiety rather than enthusiasm. It was decided that, before going public, the implementation plan should be developed to the point where it was sufficiently detailed for a realistic assessment to be made of how implementation of the IBL curriculum would affect individuals. An aggregation of individual needs helped to shape forms of mass communication that included everyone. The curriculum developers used these to keep staff and students informed of programme plans and the progress of the IBL implementation. The most effective of these methods were the notice board, newsletter, information pack and progress report.

Notice boards

The notice board is probably the most conventional and universally employed method of communicating information from the planning to the operational levels of an organization. In spite of this long tradition, its use is highly problematical even when deployed with care and conscientiously maintained. The first task is getting the notice board noticed. 'Notice boards should be installed in places where people congregate' (Andrews 1995: 58). Since students and facilitators congregate in the IBL rooms, that is an obvious place to post information of interest to those groups. A classic site for a notice board is in the entrance hall to a building frequented by the people one wishes to address. This only works if there is enough space for one or more people to stand and browse the notices. Even when the board is well sited, the notices on it can go unread if they are not well presented, relevant and topical. The design needs to be eye-catching and keywords that are significant to the targeted reader prominently displayed. The notice board should not be overcrowded with competing information and, most especially, old notices should be removed as soon as they pass their 'display until' date. There are few more off-putting and dispiriting sights than a notice board cluttered with layers of curling yellowed A4.

Location, presentation and currency may all be optimal and still the notice is ignored – some people are temperamentally drawn to notice boards whilst others will pass them by without a glance. There is always a degree of uncertainty about whether a notice has been read by all interested parties, which means it cannot be relied upon as a primary medium of communication. At APU, the notice board is used to repeat in a more permanent form, or augment with added detail, information that has already been communicated verbally.

Newsletter

In the curriculum development phase of the IBL implementation project, a precursor of the current IBL newsletter was produced each month by the Director of Studies and circulated in the health schools and practice areas. Its purpose was to educate and motivate students, academics and practitioners. It addressed the matters of most concern about IBL philosophy and methodology, such as, what it meant to the curriculum and practice experience, what effect it might have on personal and professional expectations.

Post-implementation, the primary function of the IBL newsletter is to circulate news of curriculum activities to students, practitioners and academics. Although the newsletter is physically a medium of publication – printed at the centre and distributed one-way out to its readership – it is part of the two-way traffic of information. It feeds forward fresh content about changes in strategies, policies, guidelines, roles and responsibilities – most of which comes as news to students and staff. It feeds back data that students and staff already have some knowledge of (a worm's eye view of what is going on) after it has been processed into updated forms to give the whole picture (the bird's eye view). Examples of feedback information are the project progress and performance evaluation reports.

The IBL newsletter is published once in each semester and is circulated throughout the trusts and health schools.

Great pains are taken to ensure that the editorial and production values of the IBL newsletter are comparable to those of a commercial in-house magazine. The quality of content and presentation is a subtext that assures the readership that they are worthy of respect and that their involvement is valued. Knowledge of how others are involved in other areas underlines that what is happening to individuals is a shared experience. Links are formed, interpersonal and interdisciplinary, that draw the students, academics and practitioners together in reciprocal support and common endeavour.

IBL newsletter distribution information

- To the practice areas in hospitals, community, care homes and private hospitals – via academic link lecturers – for students, practice supervisors, mentors and all practitioners.

- Via IBL facilitators – for IBL groups and display on IBL room notice boards.

- Via members of the Curriculum Management Group – comprising representatives from the five NHS trusts with nursing students at APU, the Workforce Development Confederation and field leaders – for onward circulation.

- To senior management – comprising Deans of the health schools, the Health Business Centre and the Workforce Development Confederation.

- To the admissions manager and placements manager.

Facilitators' Directory and Log

The 'Facilitators' Directory and Log' is designed as an aid to reflection (see Figure 7.1 for an example of the contents).

Facilitators are encouraged to make notes of the salient features of their personal experience and to examine in what ways the experience affected them – what learning took place and which areas require further development. The need to

Personal details
Useful contacts
Assessment of practice information
Inquiry-Based Learning principles
IBL tutorial process steps
IBL modules
Practice placements information
Roles and responsibilities
Student support
Facilitators' Log
Practice staff feedback record
Professional development and scholarly activity record
Reminders section
Notes section

Figure 7.1 Example of the content of the 'Facilitators' Directory and Log'

express their thoughts and feelings about what happened in writing imposes a formal discipline that enables the reflective process to proceed at a greater depth and with considerably more precision. It must be said, however, that some facilitators find documenting their reflections a chore from which they would rather be excused.

Nevertheless, a detailed account of the facilitator's experiences, observations and conclusions is also of value to peers and colleagues as an aid to their own reflection and learning. It is also of assistance in curriculum evaluation, and as a measure of how effectively facilitators are fulfilling their role and the areas in which further staff development would be useful.

IBL information package for practitioners

The information package comprised a comprehensive description of the IBL curriculum, together with the rationale for its introduction and a full discussion of the valuable contribution it would be making to nursing practice in future. The packages were developed and distributed – to all the practice areas to which students are allocated for their practice experience – well in advance of the scheduled implementation date of the new curriculum. This gave practitioners, particularly the practice supervisors and mentors who would be interfacing directly with students, the time and opportunity to become fully conversant with all those aspects of the IBL curriculum that would impinge on the educational responsibilities of their role. Accordingly, the package included, in addition to IBL philosophy and methodology, formal definitions of policies, procedures, guidelines, the level of students, what students can and cannot do, expectations in respect of student performance, and APU's expectations in respect of the practitioners' performance of their role as supervisors and mentors.

As with the other means of communication set up for the implementation of the IBL curriculum, the packages had a positive effect on motivation, confidence and interpersonal relationships. The links between academics and practitioners were reinforced by the inclusion of the contact details of the IBL facilitators in the package to improve liaison and support. See Figure 7.2 for the content list of the IBL information package for practitioners.

Project progress report

The project progress report was initially produced by the IBL coordinator as a project control document to give an update of the status of the development phase of the project to senior academic managers of the health schools, Workforce Development Confederation managers, managers of NHS trusts and senior administrative managers. The project's progress was also reported to academic and practice staff to keep them informed.

Post-implementation, the report evolved into an annual summary of the status of the implementation phase of the project, with an analysis of the current condition of the IBL curriculum, conclusions drawn and recommended actions for the IBL Curriculum Management Group.

CONTENTS

University contact details
Concepts and philosophies underpinning the curriculum
The Common Foundation Programme
Field Programmes

- Adult Nursing Studies
- Childhood Studies
- Mental Health Studies
- Learning Disabilities Studies

Programme structure
Semesters and modules in the curriculum
Processes of the curriculum
Practice experience
Assessment issues
Student support
Evaluation strategy

APPENDICES

Code of Professional Conduct
Outcomes to be achieved for entry to Field Programme
Competencies for entry to Register
Sample documents
Practice Assessment Record
Clinical Nursing Skills Record
Clinical Nursing Skills Workbook
Module Guides
Integration of content strands
Directory of IBL facilitators

Figure 7.2 Example of the contents of the IBL information package for practitioners

Conclusion

Effective communication about the IBL project within the health schools and trusts and beyond has been a critical factor in the successful implementation of the IBL curriculum. It has made it possible to raise the profile of the IBL philosophy and methodology and increase the awareness of the staff directly involved in the new curriculum and those looking on. The open and thorough reporting of issues and outcomes has given a high degree of credibility to the project, winning the confidence of students, practitioners and academics, and so greatly increasing staff morale and motivation. It has also enhanced the standard of internal and external communications in the pre-registration nursing programme at APU.

Chapter 8

Subproject 3: classroom compass

Introduction

'A common problem reported by staff was the difficulty of dealing with large groups and in particular encouraging student interest and involvement in large classes' (Ballantyne *et al.* 2000). IBL can address the educational problem described here, but before it can do so, something has to be done first about the material infrastructure of traditional teaching – because those large classes sit in large rooms. The move from a teacher-centred to a student-centred mode of learning is not simply philosophical, it must also be physical – from an environment designed for lecturing to large groups, to an environment designed for cooperative learning in small groups.

'School of nursing facing financial cuts' is a perennial headline and finding the funding for radical nurse education initiatives that involve wholesale change is usually an insurmountable problem, as Feletti (1993) noted. This was not the case on this occasion. APU, the Workforce Development Confederation and the local NHS trusts were able to make a budgetary provision that was sufficient to implement IBL. The author, as IBL Coordinator, was therefore in the happy position of being able to implement the various dimensions of the classroom compass from first principles – resulting in a learning environment that is highly conducive to small IBL group working.

Group arrangement

'For the greatest personal growth, it is best if [students] are assigned to the groups' (Woods 1994: 4.1). Selection makes it possible to avoid the formation of groups that are too homogeneous and therefore dull and passive. Heterogeneity offers the possibility of a clash of opposites to energize the group, sparking off new ideas and changing attitudes. That sort of variety might, on the face of it, have been difficult to achieve at APU because the pattern of IBL groups corresponds to the nursing fields – so that the groups tie in with the speciality programmes designed for professional practice. It follows that students must be allocated to their IBL groups to achieve this necessary continuity, and that is a step towards internal conformity in the groups. However, randomness in the selection, as Allen *et al.* (2001) point out, injects heterogeneity into the group. At APU, students are randomly assigned to the NHS trust sites within their nursing field – except, for example, local recruits who request an assignment near to home. This appears to reintroduce a satisfactory range of individual variation into the groups.

Group identity

The group will tend to cohere over time into a unit, although there is a good deal of variation in the degree of cohesion achieved and how long it takes. Ideally the group comes together at least well enough to have a sense of its own unique identity so that the group members can face the triumphs and vicissitudes of the programme, and of student life, together – giving and receiving mutual support and uniting their strengths in a common effort.

Being included, feeling valued, are powerful social motivators that help learners function well and learn more effectively than they would as isolated individuals. That is one of the reasons why group productivity can be greater than the total productivity of all the students working alone. It follows that anything that can be done to attract an individual into adopting the group, as Gross (1990) suggests, is worth doing. One strategy employed at APU to encourage students to commit to their IBL group is to give each group a unique identifier. Every student intake has its own category – birds, colours, trees, counties and rivers are examples. IBL facilitators choose names from the intake category for their groups. Thus in the 'Bird' intake one can find the 'Falcon', 'Heron', 'Partridge' and 'Robin' groups. This simple device is a remarkably effective way to encourage students to identify with and support the group – maximizing their own learning and the learning of the other members of the group.

Group size

'Group size usually comes down to who is available to serve as tutor, how many students there are, and how many tutors can be recruited and how many rooms located' (Wilkerson 1996: 24). This paints a picture that is probably very familiar to professional educators. It is all too often the case that the size of IBL groups is predetermined by the circumstances of real life. While there are always going to be practical limits to any human activity, occasionally something can be done by way of strategic management – forward planning, budgeting, staff development and timetabling – to change how things are, so that circumstances are not so restrictive in future. If it does prove possible to get a degree or two of freedom in the operational area, then a theoretical consideration of what group size is optimal for learning may be useful.

Phillips and Phillips (1993) classified groups by size – an 'intimate group' has two to six students, a 'small group' seven to fifteen, and if there are more than fifteen students that is a 'large group'. PBL programmes seem inclined to the belief that

FACILITATED GROUP SIZE	APPROACH	SOURCE
5 to 6	PBL	Woods 1994: 4.1
5 to 8 / 9	PBL	Barrows 1996: 5
5 to 8	PBL	Feletti 1993: 144
8 or less	PBL	Wilkerson 1996: 24
8 to 10	PBL	De Graaff 1993: 11
8 to 10	IBL	Magnussen et al. 2000: 361
15 to 20	PBL	Alavi 1995: 6
15 to 40	IBL	Feletti 1993: 144

Figure 8.1 A selection of group sizes

learning is maximized in an intimate group (see Figure 8.1). Putting such a low ceiling on the number of students working together is not regarded as desirable in IBL, which depends for much of its effectiveness upon a certain amount of pre-existing variation – in terms of backgrounds, experiences, knowledge bases and learning styles – in the students who make up the group. The differences between individuals are an asset to the group because they enlarge the total learning resource the group can call upon, and diversity is a stimulus to learning because the existence of a multiplicity of points of view means that truth of anything has to be arrived at by argument, not assumption.

In an intimate group there is liable to be a paucity of inputs from students – a shortfall which encourages over-reliance on the facilitator's store of knowledge. This leaves the group dangerously prone to becoming teacher-centred. A purely practical additional objection is that there may be too few students to carry out the many group work phases of the IBL tutorial process.

When the group is large 'group processes dominate, and individuality is sub-merged' (Phillips and Phillips 1993: 540). The interactions between a large number of people take on a socio-political dimension in which individuals with shared opinions gravitate towards one another, moving away from those who have different standpoints. If the opposing camps pull away too far a line of fracture opens up and the group splits into 'us' and 'them'. In another similarly negative scenario, the large group may turn upon and reject an idiosyncratic person whose views diverge too markedly from the norm, or, as is more likely to be the case, from the views of the more aggressive members of the group. The emergence of a small alpha group – the self-selected 'natural leaders' who dominate proceedings to the detriment of everyone else's wants and needs – is a typical phenomenon of large assemblies of people. Certainly it is the author's own experience that in a large group it is often the same few voices that are heard – some students and the lecturer doing most of the talking for the silent, uninterested, disaffected majority.

Once the many are dominated by the few, then any overt manifestation of individuality by the less assertive or articulate is suppressed, and any attempt to participate is taken as an attempt to seize power and soon thwarted. The defining dynamic of the large group is conflict – in effect it suffers from an excess of diversity. To control conflict, the organizational structure of the large group is obliged to move back towards the authoritarian model. In that return to traditional modes of teaching, student autonomy becomes increasingly compromised until a point is reached beyond which the wishes and needs of the individual can no longer be heard and all pretensions to an egalitarian philosophy of student-centred learning are extinguished.

When APU decided to move away from teaching and learning in the large groups that were normal at that time in nursing schools – one lecturer and between fifty and two hundred students were common – it settled on a preferred group size of ten to fifteen students. Groups in this range were big enough for their members to input sufficient diversity into group work for the IBL methodology to function effectively, but not so large that individual learning opportunities were unduly diminished by hostile group dynamics. It was considered that in a small group a point of balance could be achieved between the scholarly and social aspects of learning that would optimize group productivity and enhance learning.

The benefits that accrue from the one-to-many, many-to-one, social binding within a small group cannot be overemphasized. One researcher's perceptive summary is worth quoting at length – 'cooperative learning and achievement are strongly mediated by the cohesiveness of the group, in essence . . . students will help one another learn because they care about one another and want one another to succeed' (Salvin 1996: 46). As the group works together in the IBL tutorial process – exploring, reviewing, consolidating and reflecting – there are opportunities for its members to bond emotionally and psychologically. There are also opportunities for individuals to share what they have with the group, and for the group in return to ensure that no one is left out in the search for knowledge.

Ideally, within the group, collaboration and mutual understanding feed one another so they develop together in a virtuous upwards spiral. Individual differences do not divide the group, they make it stronger. Individuality is enjoyed and celebrated for its own sake and also because it excites and energizes cooperative learning. This is active learning, with immediate feedback within the group (Woods 1994). At its best, when the group gels into a close-knit team, the small group should provide the pre-registration nursing student with an authentic foretaste of what it is like to function as a member of a multiprofessional care team.

Group room

In traditional teaching, classrooms are custom-built to accommodate scores of pairs of eyes staring one way and one pair staring back. They tend therefore to be large, long and narrow – with furniture put out in a grid that means the only person able to see everyone else's face is the lecturer. None of this is of any use in IBL – indeed each one of these features would represent a fatal obstruction to the effective implementation of student-centred learning. The first sight of even an empty IBL classroom generally makes a striking impression on academic visitors to APU.

It is immediately apparent from the layout, decor, furnishings and equipment that something very different from didactic modes of education goes on in such a room. The IBL rooms at APU exemplify the principle that 'the environment in which the group works, including the room and its facilities, can have a powerful influence on how well the group functions' (Phillips and Phillips 1993: 541) – an assertion roundly echoed by Little (1998).

Frost (1996), Gibbon (1998) and Wilkie (2000) variously make the point that the first logistical requirement of student-centred approaches is a sufficiency of appropriately sized rooms. The university allocated twenty-three rooms of a size that would comfortably accommodate small groups to the IBL project – and in so doing helped to turn the possibility of a successful implementation into a probability. It was instructive to observe how as the technical redevelopment of the rooms proceeded, the initial curiosity of students and staff progressively changed to interest and, as the rooms were completed and fitted out, that interest flare into enthusiasm. The progression of the physical conversion from lecture rooms to fully customized IBL rooms was symbolic of the ideological journey of emancipation students would be making from a teacher-dominated to a student-autonomous environment. And, since an authoritarian regime constrains the freedom of educators as well as learners, it symbolized the change in role of staff, from lecturers to facilitators.

The dimensions and proportions of the IBL room are a major physical determinant of the amount and quality of personal interaction within the group. The quality of interaction in turn is a highly significant contributor to group cohesion and student motivation (Dolmans et al. 2001). The shape and size of the room are judged to be satisfactory when the group (with its facilitator) is able to arrange itself so that everyone can see everyone else – David et al. (1999). In practice this means sitting in a circle, or semicircle.

In disposing themselves about the room, the members of the group will intuitively observe the complex set of rules of social behaviour that govern such occasions. Over the millennia humans have evolved a sophisticated etiquette for use when gathering together in a group. How much personal space the assembled individuals will need depends upon the mix of sex, age and class – the usual suspects – as mediated by the micro and macro cultural norms of those present. As long as the group is close enough to read facial expression and body language easily – but not too close for emotional and psychological comfort – and the group feels neither cramped nor dwarfed by the room then students and facilitator will be able to interact productively.

The emotional and psychological climate of the group is likely to be affected by the colours used to decorate the IBL room – which are pale green and lilac at APU. We cannot pretend that the choice of these particular colours was based on a body of sound research about the influence of colour on learning – the impetus was more artistic than scientific. However, a lay appreciation is that greens are restful and violets promote reflection and meditation. Pale shades have been used in the main rather than raw hues so if the colours do have a positive effect, it will be a gentle and unobtrusive one.

Each IBL room is equipped with an overhead projector, whiteboard, flipcharts, notice boards and other visual aids and facilities. Less conventionally, every room also has a television, video recorder and filing cabinet. A computer provides local word processing and graphics and remote access to APU intranet resources such as WebCT and the university library, and via the Internet to other academic and professional resources.

The students' chairs are to a special ergonomic design that allows them to dispense with desks – a writing slab is simply swung into position for note-taking. Otherwise the students and facilitator can pull the chairs into the informal circle that is optimal for IBL interpersonal communication. No person – especially not those with a functional role in the tutorial process, the chair, scribe and facilitator – is more or less important in the group than anyone else. Setting, group size and physical positioning strongly reinforce behaviour that is both independent and sharing – a potent psychosocial synthesis of the logical opposites, autonomy and mutuality.

Psychologically, the group 'owns' the room and its contents – with the facilitator as co-learner. Whatever the group's academic reason for coming to the room, its interactions in the IBL tutorial process create a social climate that fosters interpersonal skills, as Maitland and Cowdray (2001) reported. From the theoretical perspective, the classroom compass can also be considered as a part of a meta-learning control loop. It is a given that the sensory and psychosocial 'landscape' of the IBL room exerts an influence on group and individual learning behaviours. When students learn new ways of learning, by observing and participating in the learning of others, metalearning takes place. As a consequence, the psychosocial – and the sensory too if the group makes changes in the physical environment – landscape alters. The new landscape exerts a different influence on learning behaviours and the metalearning control loop begins another iteration.

Group work schedule

'Task boundaries prevent the group from following non-constructive paths and protect individuals from inappropriate activities by the group' (Phillips and Phillips 1993: 541). The point being made is that student autonomy is not synonymous with student anarchy. The IBL group has objectives which it is unlikely to achieve if it conducts itself in a random, unfocused way. The absence of a guiding structure is as bad as the authoritarian alternative of too much control being exerted from outside the group. The well considered timetable starts with a fair estimate of what can be expected from a group – taking into account the real-life limitations of accommodation, time availability and productivity – to schedule group tutorials and individual activities in ways that maximize learning. When developed by an experienced planner, the timetable does not constrain the creativity of the autonomous learner.

One defining difference between the IBL timetable and a traditional one is in the treatment of self-directed study. In the latter, the days are given over to classroom sessions. By default, studying by oneself or 'doing your homework with a friend' is confined to the evenings and weekends. Self-directed learning in an IBL curriculum is not a second-best marginalized learning activity. It occupies centre stage and is regarded as being of first importance.

In the timetable developed at APU, the five steps of the tutorial process are distributed across an entire semester period. In this model, the extensive inter-tutorial step gaps that are left are occupied by, mainly, clinical practice experience, skills development sessions in the skills laboratory and by self-directed study activities. The latter activities are formally scheduled so that students have educational prime time in which to explore information resources, reflect on learning issues, prepare for the next tutorial step, or consolidate the last by tidying up loose threads of inquiries.

Some of the time students will work alone, sometimes in twos or threes, or in the full IBL group with or without the facilitator. Non-facilitated IBL group time is formally scheduled so that students can work completely independently of their facilitator. No matter how able the facilitator, how light the touch of the guiding hand, in the final analysis the facilitator is not a student – with the group, of course, but never truly one of the group. In the absence of the facilitator, the non-facilitated group can take cooperative learning a stage further. The group members can be even more forthcoming in discussion and review of their individual and group learning needs and issues; and in devising and agreeing the group work plan, they are able to practise organizational and other management skills. Thus scheduled self-directed learning sessions cover the whole gamut of educational possibility. Independent work has a beneficial effect on the individual's confidence level and self-esteem whilst the group sessions exercise interpersonal skills, reinforce social ties and promote communal well-being.

There are three other timetabled activities. Resource sessions are delivered by a subject expert (who might be an invited speaker) to clarify concepts, offer concentrated additional information or, by creating a change of mode and pace, to act as a stimulus to learning. A fixed resource session is one that all students are encouraged to attend. A variant is the parallel resource session. As the name suggests, two or more of these sessions are run at the same time, each offering a different insight into the same module topic and scenario concepts. The IBL group elects one or two students to attend each parallel resource session to represent the rest of the group. The representatives write summary reports to share with the IBL group in the next non-facilitated IBL group tutorial. This strategy adds another dimension to the learning experience since the representatives have to accept responsibility for the IBL group's learning as well as their own. This activity is very similar in concept and execution to what students do for the IBL review tutorial.

Clinical nursing skills laboratory sessions and clinical practice placements, which both aim to integrate theory and practice, are the remaining scheduled learning experiences. These three activities, with the tutorial process and the various study sessions, make up the varied learning strategies that are deployed selectively in the IBL curriculum to help each individual student attain their own specific learning outcomes.

Clinical nursing skills laboratory

Everything that a nursing student learns eventually leads, directly or indirectly, to the giving of client/patient care. This involves, though it is by no means limited to, the adept performance of a variety of clinical skills. The process of acquiring these skills starts at the very beginning of, and continues throughout, the pre-registration nursing programme. Since it is a giant step from the intellectual contemplation in the IBL room of how the needs of a theoretical client/patient might best be met, to a confrontation with the living and breathing actuality in the clinical area, an intermediate learning experience is provided by way of the clinical nursing skills laboratories. There are three such at APU, each containing an array of multi-media and audiovisual learning resources, as well as computer access to the Internet, a hardcopy library of nursing texts, and digital film-making equipment.

The skills laboratories are fully resourced and equipped as standard patient care areas with replicated nursing stations. The 'patients' in this realistic environment are made-for-purpose mannequins and models, and, when appropriate, the students themselves – the latter occasions providing a valuable learning experience from a client/patient perspective. A credible scenario is the starting point. With the help of facilitators, skills laboratory coaches and demonstrators, the students practise their basic nursing skills in a risk-free environment.

The semester-specific clinical nursing skills workbook contains prompts or triggers for each skill that help the student recall and reflect upon their performance and perceptions of care. Skills that a student has already learned and rehearsed are logged in a clinical nursing skills record. A student will also maintain a portfolio of performance and professional development. This is a further aid to reflection and self-assessment. It is also a resource for assigned work and evidence of their acquisition of appropriate personal and professional attributes.

Assessment process

A move from a teacher-centred to student-centred curriculum 'requires rethinking how to assess student learning in such an environment' (Duch and Groh 2001: 95). As a matter of simple academic survival, the student will allocate most study time and attention to those elements of the curriculum on which the student will be assessed. In recognition of this pragmatism, we took care at APU in developing our assessment methods for the IBL curriculum that they should reflect as far as possible IBL philosophy and closely model the IBL dimensions of learning outcomes, that is, focused on the concept knowledge base, clinical reasoning skills, interpersonal attributes, clinical skills and self-directed study.

The assessment procedures selected and developed are designed to reflect the integrated approach of IBL and the holistic nature of nursing at its best. They include:

- group presentation
- care study

- reflective case study
- critical incident analysis
- evaluation of a care package
- concept map poster forum.

These assessments take place at the end of each module throughout the three-year pre-registration nursing programme. They require the student to integrate appropriate knowledge and skills, demonstrating their application in practice. The assessments are linked by their specific learning outcomes to the programme's broader competencies, which in turn link directly to the curriculum profile of the registered nurse.

However, APU is not the final arbiter of the assessment process. The statutory bodies impose assessment procedures that largely test the student's capacity for the recall of discrete items of knowledge. The IBL students are therefore obliged to undertake one formal written examination during the three-year programme – an inappropriate method of assessment in the circumstances, as Walton and Matthews (1989) remarked.

Evaluation strategy

'Evaluation is concerned more fundamentally with deciding on the value or "worthwhileness" of a learning process as well as the effectiveness with which it is being carried out' (Lawton 1981: 147). It is impossible to overstress the importance of having an evaluation strategy that can determine value and effectiveness when one is implementing a whole curriculum that is so new, and so radically different in its philosophy and methodology, that there is no prior academic or practitioner experience of working with it to hand – neither institutionally nor individually. Of course this means that a new evaluation strategy has to be developed and implemented as well, because when what is being done changes then how it is measured must change too.

By definition, evaluation is an after-the-event activity, but that does not mean it can be put to one side for later – it has to be taken into consideration from the outset of the development phase, because the data requirements of the evaluation strategy form part of the design brief for the curriculum. Once the curriculum is implemented, the evaluation results are fed back to control the operation. Provided learning and other outcomes are being satisfactorily achieved then no corrective action by management is necessary. If the results show some aspect of the curriculum is not being implemented effectively then the causes need to be found and remedial changes made in methods or human/material resources.

The Curriculum Management Group (CMG) brings together representatives of the health schools, Workforce Development Confederation and the participating health care trusts to monitor and evaluate the IBL curriculum. An IBL evaluator was appointed to initiate and coordinate the evaluation strategy early in the project. Later, a research assistant was recruited and dedicated to the IBL curriculum.

METHODS	TARGET GROUP	ADDITIONAL DATA COLLECTION AND ANALYSIS
1 Questionnaires: • recruitment and selection processes • the Induction programme • end of module • end of semester	• students • IBL facilitators • clinical practice supervisors • student facilitators (practice)	• attrition rate • student progression • assessment results • student attendance • completion of the programme
2 Interviews/consultation groups: • end of year		

Figure 8.2 Schematic overview of the evaluation process

Evaluation affects everyone who is involved in any way with the curriculum, because directly or indirectly it measures everyone's performance – not just that of students, academics and practitioners but also of managers, administrators and other staff providing services. Not all of these are formally measured, but those that are, need the assurance that the procedures are consistent, reliable and valid. The process should also be demonstrably beneficial to those being evaluated. Normally, this is realized by making sure the evaluation results are fed back to the originators of the data, so they can use it to improve their performance.

The APU evaluation process is based upon questionnaires and interviews (see Figure 8.2 for a schema of the process).

Evaluation methodology

The IBL evaluator prepares reports for:

• CMG members
• IBL facilitators – to share with their students
• module leaders
• set coordinators.

The report is also published in the biannual IBL newsletter, which is distributed throughout the IBL community.

The CMG has been able to make changes in operational procedures and staff development as appropriate in response to feedback received in this way from students, practitioners, academics and others – in a reasonable timescale. It is beyond the author's remit and the scope of this book to give a detailed account of the actual curriculum evaluation results and how feedback affects the operation of the IBL programme.

Conclusion

At APU, the classroom compass is a range of activities, processes and structures that conform to the tenets of student-centred learning in general and IBL in particular. The components of the classroom compass have been designed specifically to work separately and in concert to maximize each student's learning experiences whether self-directed or cooperative within the small group.

Chapter 9

Subproject 4: practice experience

Introduction

Nursing is a vocation that is practised. The student's experiences in practice – in the clinical setting – are therefore a necessary component of an educational programme for which the eventual culmination is a professionally qualified registered nurse. Accordingly, the United Kingdom Central Council (UKCC) (1999) recommends that practice should have an equal weighting to theory – 50 per cent each. Practice is not something that only starts when nurse education ends, as Creedy *et al.* (1992) confirmed, but rather it progresses hand in hand with theory throughout the programme.

At APU, a new intake of IBL students will have their first direct experiences in the practice setting within five weeks of their commencement – implementing the United Kingdom Central Council (UKCC 1999: 29) recommendation 'to ensure that practice skills and placements are introduced at an early stage in the programme'. Students will already have anticipated this event to some extent because from its very outset the IBL pre-registration nursing programme is one that promotes 'learning which can be transferred to and integrated with a number of clinical situations' (Cooke 1995: 104). This it does in part by having realistic scenarios for students to work with in the IBL tutorial process and by their participation in other practice-focused activities, most especially skills development in the IBL clinical practice skills laboratory.

A range of clinical learning experiences available in the IBL curriculum will be discussed in the remainder of this chapter under the headings of:

- identification of practice placements for student experience
- student support in the practice setting
- role of the IBL facilitator
- student reflection time in the practice setting.

Identification of practice placements for student experience

'Clinical experiences provide opportunities for students to learn about what nurses do in diverse practice environments' (Royle *et al.* 2001: 241). Unfortunately, actual practice experience is not invariably as educationally rewarding for students as it might be. 'Many student nurses find they do not know what task they should be doing during their clinical placements' (Willis 1996: 55). This was a recognized problem in the diploma level programme in Project 2000, where uncertainty about exactly what should be expected of students in the practice environment could be ascribed to not having programme-wide standards. The situation prompted the recommendation in 'Fitness for Practice' (UKCC 1999) that nurse education programmes should be practice-driven so that, on registration, the newly qualified practitioners will have all the skills they need to deliver safe and competent care. From the educationalist's point of view, that level of knowledge and skill can be best achieved by ensuring that the student placements for practice-based experience are scheduled at a time and place that allows what has been learned in theory to be put into practice with least delay.

The ideal practice experience for the student nurse is one that is a near-replication of scenarios that have been studied recently in the IBL tutorial process and the clinical nursing skills laboratory. When the practice follow-through is immediate and relevant, direct live action fills the theoretical, or better the virtual, framework of academically acquired knowledge with vividly unforgettable multidimensioned experiential content. Such high quality learning experiences: build practitioner levels of competence, easily and speedily; generate the true self-confidence that comes from taking effective action in situations in which the stakes are high and the consequences, for student, patient/client and those around them, are real – possibly even irreversible.

An effective integrating link between theory and practice is made by identifying the practice setting which potentially offers clinical experiences that closely correspond with the learning outcomes of modules being studied. The anticipated quality of those clinical experiences – from an educational point of view – and the current levels of understanding and competence of the student, are other important parameters that should be taken into account in the process of selecting suitable practice settings for student placements.

APU, in collaboration with the Workforce Development Confederation and local NHS trusts provides both main core and associate core placements. Main core placements are those sited in the student's 'home base' – a location, group or person, to which or to whom the student is permanently attached. As an example, in the adult nursing studies field this might be a certain area in a hospital, such as a medical, surgical or elderly care ward, or an individual professional. Students are scheduled to spend a year in each speciality to complete all three main core placements. By contrast, there is a network of associate core placements which are of short duration and scheduled to give the student an opportunity to gain experience in an area of particular interest or of educational benefit – for example, two weeks' attachment to a specialist nurse. The operational logistics of the scheduled main core and associate core placements are the responsibility of the practice placements department. A non-scheduled network of opportunistic placements also exists in which arrangements are made bilaterally at the local level, mainly for follow-up visits to areas like occupational therapy or perhaps a rehabilitation centre.

In the modular system through which the IBL curriculum is delivered, students, academics and practitioners are provided with clear guidelines about module learning outcomes and the achievements looked for in the related practice placements. The nursing field leaders and programme planners, in collaboration with the practice placements department, identify the practice settings that best fit the needs of the overall learning outcomes. The IBL students are able to exercise a degree of autonomy once in placement by negotiating their own individual learning outcomes – within the overarching module expectations – their choices being formalized in the learning contract. A wider autonomy becomes possible in the option modules made available in the students' final year where they are able to choose the practice setting and select their practice learning experiences.

Aspirations to integrate theory into practice effectively – resulting in knowledge-able and skilled practitioners – are blighted, sometimes almost confounded, by a predicament that has been bluntly summarized as 'too many students and not enough placements' (White et al. 1993). A situation exacerbated on one side by Government exhortations to increase student nurse numbers (National Health Service Executive 1998) and on the other by competition for the same fixed resources from other health care programmes. There is a limit to the number of IBL students who can be accommodated in any one practice setting at any one time. Once there are too many students for the available practitioners to guide, then the quality of learning falls away – rapidly followed by the goodwill and motivation of those practitioners.

The nursing field leaders, in collaboration with module leaders and practitioners, take pains to ensure that module outcomes are concise and unambiguous – to maximize learning in the practice setting. Additionally, much can be done by practitioner and academic managers to make the most of what placement capacity there is by cooperating to devise and implement imaginative and considered placement strategies – such as negotiating with competitor health care programmes to agree a collaborative strategy of reciprocal placements.

Student support in the practice setting

Fitness for Practice (United Kingdom Central Council 1999) recommends that support for the learning of students in practice placements should be the joint responsibility of the service providers and the higher education institutions. Reason suggests, and common sense confirms, that by acting in concert, the nursing service and nurse education can deliver all the support, guidance and supervision that students need to acquire the knowledge, skills and competencies of the professional nurse practitioner. However, the historic actuality is that the working relationship between these two natural partners has often been less than harmonious. Any such disunity inevitably de-optimizes the practice placement learning experience. As Jones (1985: 350) discovered, 'many of the faults in the clinical learning experience of nursing students . . . arise from the distancing of nurse education from nursing practice'.

There are other difficulties that can adversely affect the performance of students on placement. Most of these come about because of the nature of the practice area. Its function is patient/client care and it is geared towards that purpose and so has features that may make it from time to time incompatible with learning. For example, the often sudden extemporary nature of health care, its labour intensity, frequent staffing problems, twenty-four hours a day/seven days a week shift patterns, and so on. Add to this agitated mix the nurse lecturers, who were unsure of their role and who spent a mere half-hour a week in the wards – as related by Payne *et al.* (1991, cited by Rogers 1995).

When students are not supported in their learning in practice settings, as described above, it is an educational calamity. If IBL students are to learn effectively and productively they need to work within guidelines, their work needs to be monitored, the learning process needs to be evaluated, and what students have learned needs to be assessed. None of this happens if the IBL methodology, and as importantly its philosophy, stops at the door of the classroom. Standards and consistency and continuity are all. Students cannot be expected to be active, engaged and supported in the IBL room and passive, sidelined and neglected when they move to the clinical setting.

At APU there are a number of key operatives responsible for ensuring that the student learning experience in the practice setting is linked to theory, that the IBL approach is supported, and that the IBL programme standards are maintained. There are IBL facilitators and link tutors – who are academics – with IBL practice

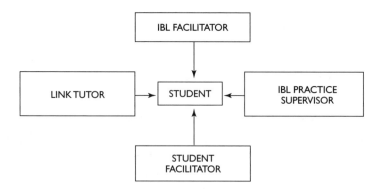

Figure 9.1 Student support mechanisms – role relationships

supervisors and student facilitators – who are practice-based (see Figure 9.1). Between them, they offer the student cohort academic, practice and personal support. They are multipurpose resources: guides and counsellors, mentors and monitors, coaches and cheerleaders. They are a collection of interrelated roles, all of which 'are needed to create the full range of educational support for practice education' (Day *et al*. 1998: 6).

Although an academic, the IBL facilitator's role – as a collaborator in the learning process with a group of students – extends into the clinical setting whenever the IBL group is scheduled for practice placement. The process of facilitation continues by guiding students in the relation of learning gained experientially back to concepts learned in the IBL room, and by helping students to develop appropriate strategies of exploration, self-directed learning, review and consolidation to engage successfully with the module scenario.

The IBL facilitator – who is also personal and academic tutor to the IBL group – will visit first year students in the practice setting once in every four weeks. Thereafter, the increasing autonomy of the students makes regular direct support of their learning a less frequent necessity. However, the IBL facilitator – as academic tutor – will still monitor student progress and will also continue to visit to discharge pastoral responsibilities as personal tutor.

The link tutor is responsible for maintaining a link between the APU health schools and their practice link areas designated for student placements. They contribute to student learning in placement and liaise with practice staff and academic staff – IBL facilitators and personal tutors.

The practice supervisor – a nurse practitioner – supports and guides students through a core placement, acts as role model, assesses student competence in practice and monitors progress, acts as a resource person on matters relating to the module scenario, fosters multidisciplinary working, and liaises with academic staff.

The practice-based student facilitator – a registered nurse – liaises with and supports students, practice supervisors and others in the implementation of IBL in the practice setting, liaises and collaborates with academic staff in the IBL curriculum, and conducts surgeries for IBL students.

Student reflection time in the practice setting

Reflection is a commonplace cognitive activity – mulling over events, reliving what one felt and thought at the time, attributing motives, drawing conclusions – anyone can do it. It is, however, a very powerful tool when used deliberately, without prejudgement, to extract meaning from one's experience of events. It often helps, when one is trying to find connections and gain an understanding of events, to get a different perspective by consulting a colleague or one of the supporting staff mentioned earlier. The need to express oneself coherently to another person often helps to make sense of one's impressions and to internalize new ideas. Reflection is the essence of critical thinking and consequently a necessary step in the process of self-directed learning. 'If students do not think reflectively about their performance their experience is incomplete, and it is unlikely that there will be relevant transfer' (Fogarty 1997: 132).

Throughout their practice placement students are encouraged to engage in the purposive reflection that leads to deep learning. In recognition of its role in IBL, 45 minutes of each day spent in the practice area are scheduled for reflection. Obviously in the clinical environment it is not always convenient to stop for a lengthy period of reflection so students make a note of anything new or unusual that occurs – to think about later when the moment, surroundings and mood are more conducive to reflection.

The need for students to reflect is a constant theme in the IBL curriculum. It begins in the IBL tutorial process and continues in their practice placements. Students continually demonstrate their reflective capabilities in individual and group work – including discussion, experiential activities, maintaining a portfolio and undertaking assignments.

Conclusion

In the IBL pre-registration nursing programme the 'application of knowledge occurs in a variety of practice settings from the classroom and lab to in-patients and community settings' (Cannon and Schell 2001: 165). However, imaginative and creative management is needed to overcome endemic shortages in the provision of practice areas suitable for student placements. Once in the clinical area, student learning is supported by a variety of practitioners and academics – who ensure that there is continuity and consistency in the use of the IBL process. In that regard, there is a constant emphasis on the rewards that the student gains from purposive reflection, namely 'new perspectives on experience and . . . the possibility of changing behaviour' (Coles 1998: 321).

Chapter 10

Subproject 5: documentation

Introduction

In the delivery of any curriculum, documentation has an educative and an administrative management function. The educative function is that it helps to organize the content and quality of the curriculum's product – which is education. The administrative function is to organize the content and quality of the means of production – which are manpower, money, materials and management. As a consequence of frequent productivity initiatives – often government inspired – that either directly affect, or have a knock-on effect upon, nurse education, changes to the means of production and therefore to the administrative documentation that models it for organizational purposes, are common. But when the IBL curriculum was introduced, it changed everything because the content and quality of the product had to alter – as well as the way in which it was produced. Thus much of the educative and administrative documentation used to manage the superseded teacher-centred educational system became either obsolete or redundant. New methods to deliver the IBL curriculum meant that new documents had to be devised, and old ones reinvented if possible or else discarded. Every rewrite of the documentation is a remodelling of the entire system of organizing the daily activities of academic and administrative staff and students – with all that this entails in terms of numbers of people, multiplicity of functions and complexity of linkages. It was the contemplation of the magnitude of this task that prompted the nomination of documentation as an IBL implementation subproject in its own right.

Because documentation is a model of the operational system, it follows that small errors at the planning stage of the documentation subproject might have unforeseen consequences in the implemented system. Those unintended repercussions might be very large since mighty oaks from little acorns grow. As Chase (1991) found – looking at work done by the management consultants and accountants Coopers & Lybrand Deloitte – up to 70 per cent of eventual production costs are predetermined by decisions made at the design stage. And if this is the cost of getting things right – what must the on-cost of getting things wrong be like?

Fortunately, there are several factors that work together in a synergistic fashion to help to reduce the risk of large errors being made in planning the design and production of documentation. First, the cost of publishing and distributing documentation in any medium – though especially for anything paper-based – is so high that it forms a highly visible item of budgetary expenditure. This means that all those whose budgets are likely to be affected will want to have a say in what is being planned.

Second, simply because the documentation of a whole operation is so complex a large number of potential users will be caught up in the planning process because their specialist knowledge is a necessary input to document design – indeed it is desirable that they themselves draft the design of the documentation they will be expected to use. The scrutiny of these intended users of the documents is of particular value because it is directed into the planning process from every quarter of the institution – a multiple viewpoint that represents an organization-wide spectrum of professional experience and operational know-how.

Third, it is a characteristic of documentation that it is not possible to decide in advance whether or not a document is going to work until it is complete in every particular. Because the design has to be done at the lowest level of detail, the designer has to think deeply about what is wanted, and express it with clarity so that the control or informational aspects of the document can be readily understood by the intended user. As a further bonus, the designed document, precisely because everything on it has had to be spelt out, is thereby rendered fully transparent – and so openly exposed to review, criticism and amendment by others.

Lastly, documents are most usually shared by two or more users. Since one person's outputs are somebody else's inputs, this means that every user reviewing the document is either assessing the quality of what the person before has done, or anticipating what the next person needs, or both. When two or more reviewers are involved in the same element of design then the probability of detecting errors is dramatically improved. This powerful constraint on faults getting through the design process will be further reinforced, it is assumed, because the users will be from different backgrounds and have different skills and so can in effect between them triangulate the error and eliminate it.

There are, naturally, factors that adversely affect the success of the documentation design and production planning process. The involvement of a relatively large number of people greatly increases the potential for disagreement between them. There may be differences of opinion about content, layout, frequency of issue, distribution, and so on. If differences are reconciled – so that everyone wins – then different views can become a positive factor. If differences can only be resolved by compromise – so nobody wins – then the quality of the documentation system may be impaired and on implementation it might be less effective.

Ironically, the high cost of producing documents can force their cost up even higher. Anxiety to avoid costly errors can result in a standard of quality so high, it far exceeds that needed for fitness for purpose. Pareto's law (Beer 1979) – also known as the 80/20 law – operates in matters of quality as it does with other aspects of production. Broadly speaking: for the first 20 per cent of the cost, one can achieve an 80 per cent quality level. This means the last 20 per cent of quality accounts for

80 per cent of the cost. The implication is that very high levels of quality are very expensive. The money wasted cannot be spent on something else so there is an opportunity cost too – the things that could have been done, but which can not be done now, because the money has been spent on excessive quality.

People resources are constrained in any event. The most active people in the management and operation of the curriculum – the key staff – make an important contribution in planning the design and production of documentation. But they are most likely the very people who are least available. So the final major constraint on the successful implementation of a new documentation system is that there is a finite amount of time that key staff can make available for creating, reviewing, testing and producing documents.

Finally, contemplation of the full range of documentation intended for use in the new IBL curriculum and a forecast of the very high set-up and maintenance costs likely to be incurred prompted a careful examination of the feasibility of transferring as much as possible to alternative media. Accordingly the benefits and costs of moving from a paper-based to an electronic-based information system were investigated (see Chapter 11).

Documents

A variety of documentation has been developed for use in the IBL curriculum (see Figure 10.1 for a selection of current documentation).

Roles within the design and production team

Because the implementation project involved the replacement of the whole curriculum by one with fundamentally different concepts and means of delivery, there was a much larger design and production team than would be needed to update a conventional programme. The principal roles are shown in Figure 10.2.

The identification of experienced authors, or volunteers willing to acquire the requisite writing and publishing skills, is a first consideration. For example, all academic staff who are module leaders – or who have at some time undertaken the role – would be conversant with the process of developing a module guide from inception to final draft.

The module leader – working to general guidelines issued by the IBL coordinator – produces the first draft of the module guide for presentation to the module leaders' team meeting for review. This is not a management meeting – its function is quality assurance. It is coordinated by someone who possesses in-depth experience of both the administrative and content background – usually this is the field leader. The procedure adopted is the peer review in which the draft module guide is subjected to an inspection process by a number of reviewers. Errors, omissions and deviations from guidelines count as quality defects. The main output of the process is a list of agreed defects and an associated action list. The module leader as author of the document is responsible for the follow-up of the action list. Another draft, free of

DOCUMENT	DESCRIPTION
Facilitators' Handbook	Defines the knowledge and skills needed by facilitators to fulfil their role. The scope of the handbook reinforces the notion of expanding definitions of the IBL curriculum, its implementation, and the role of the facilitator. The handbook is divided into sections including: • Philosophy and principles underpinning the curriculum • Programme structure and the student experience, e.g. modules, curriculum themes and strands • Processes of the curriculum, e.g. IBL process steps, roles and responsibilities within the IBL group • Assessment of theory and practice, e.g. strategy and schedule • Practice experience
Facilitators' Directory and Log	Facilitators are encouraged to think about what they are doing as well as doing it. The Directory and Log assist facilitators in reflecting on where they have come from and plan where they are going
Facilitators' Induction Programme Guide for students	Ideas to stimulate learners. Gives facilitators guidance for a variety of warm-up exercises. The booklet is also a facilitator resource that includes administrative and educational communication and areas of support for students
Students' Practice Assessment record	For assessment of practice learning. Specific learning outcomes and competencies for registration as a nurse are identified
Students' Module Guide	The module guide is intended as a source of definition and reference for a module. It includes sections on: • Learning outcomes • Scenario and core concepts • Assessment requirements • References and resources lists
Students' Clinical Nursing Skill Workbook	Provides students with a set of hands-on ideas and skills for the module being studied – to enable them to give the level of holistic and individualized care expected at their stage in the programme
IBL Information Package for Practitioners	Intended to enable practice staff to develop an understanding of the IBL curriculum, especially as it applies to the student experience in the practice areas. It includes sections on: • Concepts and philosophies underpinning IBL curriculum • Module information • Practice assessment issues • Student Portfolio guidelines • Learning contracts for students • Contact names and phone numbers of IBL facilitators and link tutors

Figure 10.1 Examples of current documents in the IBL curriculum

ROLE	RESPONSIBILITY
Author	Field leaders, module leaders, skills laboratory coordinator, subject leaders
Editor and standards coordination	IBL coordinator
Production administration	IBL administrator

Figure 10.2 Principal roles in document design and production

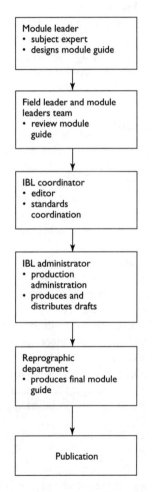

Figure 10.3 Design and production processes in the first eighteen months of implementation

the previously identified defects, is re-presented to the module leaders' meeting for review. There may be several iterations of the peer review process. When a final error-free draft is agreed, copies are sent to the field leader and IBL coordinator for ratification.

As editor in this case, the IBL coordinator checks the finished text, for example for stylistic errors and conformity to guidelines. From the early stages of the project up to eighteen months after implementation the IBL coordinator worked closely with module leaders to introduce and maintain an IBL house style to give module guides a uniform look and language, to make them more readily accessible to students and other users (see Figure 10.3).

The production administration role is taken by the IBL administrator who is responsible for the desk-top publishing of the final definitive draft and its distribution to the relevant members of the design and production team. The role also involves liaising with the reprographic department to prepare master copies of high volume documents – such as module guides.

The production schedule

The efficient publishing and distribution of large numbers of different documents, often in high volumes, relies upon quite tight scheduling at every step of the production process. Constrained resources – especially reprographic – mean that every production run is time contingent. There is little or no scope to introduce time allowances and consequently any slippage tends to result in missed deadlines and potentially missed due dates. Often it seems that the only certainty in the process is that everything takes longer than estimated.

The main protection from the threat of delay is to start the whole process as early as possible. Ample time in which to complete the intermediate steps leading up to the due date make it possible to set realistic goals for those responsible for each step. The production schedule is made known to everyone involved for accommodation in their own timetables. However, there are limits on the use of this strategy. If production times are too extended, there is more opportunity for changes to occur in the operational area. The curriculum and how it is delivered are subject to a greater or lesser degree of adjustment – especially in the early months of implementation. Because there is constant change, the document developer is sometimes trying to hit a moving target and an overly extended production time makes this more difficult.

Quality control

Because we were creating a documentation system from scratch for the entirely new IBL curriculum, there were no existing templates or examples on which to base the document designs. All the initial design work had to be done in the abstract. Once we had our first tangible product – the final draft of a module guide – we became more confident of our capacity to produce documents that conformed to the standards of quality we had set for ourselves, and which had a house style that was attractive and distinctive.

Producing the first document helped to develop and test procedures for quality assurance (the pre-production checks) and quality control (the checks made post-production). These procedures were further developed to create a system for coordinating quality maintenance and quality improvement in the implemented IBL curriculum.

Conclusion

Because documentation is the means by which the delivery of the IBL curriculum is controlled and informed, any level of quality less than 'fit for purpose' potentially threatens the viability of the IBL implementation project. Our experience at APU shows that it is possible for a core team comprising academics, the IBL coordinator and administration staff, aided by a wider community of potential users, to design, produce and maintain a range of high quality documents to meet the diverse needs of the IBL pre-registration nursing programme.

Chapter 11

Subproject 6:
electronic resources

Introduction

Nowadays, to show surprise at the extent to which the computer has infiltrated every aspect of Western life is to show one's age. The current generation of students entering schools of nursing is only startled when something that plainly should be, is not computerized. Computerization in post-industrial societies seems to be an autocatalytic process. That is, information technology (IT) functionality increases the volume and complexity of information so that a further investment in IT capacity becomes necessary to manage it, and the cycle starts a new iteration.

Certainly the professional nurse must be competent in IT to practise effectively in the modern care environment and for that reason alone nursing students should be skilled in the use of computers – 'meeting the practice requirements of pre-registration programmes might be better achieved by more widespread, planned use of information technology' (United Kingdom Central Council 1999: 41). The other reason is that the acquisition of the large body of knowledge students must have for graduation and registration is far more efficiently accomplished when it is computer-aided.

The 'Dearing Report' (Dearing 1997), talking of higher education institutions in general, envisaged the onward development and integration of electronic sources of information in the teaching and learning of students. This movement can be readily observed at APU in the pre-registration nursing IBL curriculum with the substantial migration of information from its traditional paper source to an electronic one – completed in October 2002.

Naturally enough such a revolutionary move calls for school-wide planning and coordination; translation of documents to online formats; reorientation of student and staff to the use of IT; explanatory and advisory communications with and between students and staff; troubleshooting support for technical problems; and academic and administrative staff development. The strategy also relies upon not inconsiderable IT hardware and software costs. The primary justification for the upheaval, effort and investment in resources involved is threefold: cost, convenience and flexibility. The greater cost-effectiveness and practicality of electronic-based information is apparent when one compares the relative costs, convenience and flexibility of updating a single record on a database with printing and distributing hundreds of copies of the same information on paper.

The educative process that takes place between educator and student (and between student and student in IBL) comprises information processing, interaction and communication. Traditionally these subprocesses have been conducted either face-to-face or mediated, most often, by paper. The migration away from paper-based information means that, in future, many such educator/student mediations will be performed via the computer. The technology that makes this not just a reality but a very significant educational advance in its own right is WebCT (Web Course Tools). WebCT is being implemented at various institutions in the United Kingdom (Communication and Information Technology Services 2001). Pre-registration nursing programme WebCT has been adopted as a mandatory information tool in the APU health schools for every intake of students – to make actual their androgogic status as adult learners who are responsible for their own learning (Knowles 1990).

Computers in IBL rooms

If students are to be relying to a significant extent on electronic-based information, it follows that there must be sufficient terminals and workstations to meet demand so that access does not become an issue. That is not average demand, but demand when it is at or near its peak – ensuring timely access to a terminal being analogous to ensuring that every student has the key texts when they need them. Putting computers in the IBL rooms makes for ready access and therefore greater use which, in turn, enhances learning (Bignell *et al.* 2001). A further facility is the computer laboratory where students can access the full range of communication tools: email, electronic conferencing, word processing and Web access to their programme materials and other resources.

Of particular importance in the IBL context is that 'computers can perform functions that are helpful to groups' (Phillips and Phillips 1993: 547). This may be as simple as displaying material – such as a scenario – which the group can refer to in discussion. It can be used to produce instant summaries of the contents of the whiteboard or flipchart for group members to take away to support their own notes. Email, messaging and chat rooms can keep the group in touch with one another's explorations in self-directed learning, or can be used by a few students with a shared interest who want to carry on with a minor line of inquiry that is not central to the group's purpose.

There is only a very narrow range of human behaviour that is of any utility when interacting with a computer, namely: keying, using the mouse, watching the screen, perhaps listening, loading and unloading disks and CDs. Consequently when seated in front of the computer, the dominant extrovert tends to become quieter and more patient, the shy introvert, more active and positive. Intra-group communication may be improved as a result of the computer's moderating influence and, in turn, the creative functioning of the group enhanced. Computers can occasionally be a distraction – sidetracking the group into interesting but unproductive areas – but on balance 'the positive aspects of computers, along with their superior ability to handle information can be used to enhance the capabilities of both facilitator and group' (Phillips and Phillips 1993: 547).

Move from paper-based to electronic-based information

At APU, the plan to migrate from paper-based to mainly electronic-based information was implemented over a twelve-month period, in three stages – developing awareness, staff and student development, ongoing support (see Figure 11.1).

The Workforce Development Confederation and NHS trust colleagues were strongly supportive of the move, provided always that the quality of the electronic-based information would be comparable to the quality that had been customarily achieved for paper-based information. Practice and academic staff were reasonably certain that the IT skills of students would improve dramatically once students came to rely routinely upon accessing a computer to enter, store and retrieve their IBL programme information. Nor did staff feel that students would be deprived of

STAGE   **STRATEGY**

1   Develop awareness and understanding of the rationale and process for the change:

- Provide recruitment information pack
- Inform current students of the change
- Include the transition topic as an agenda item in meetings involving students, such as field committee meetings
- Display awareness information about the change on TV screens
- Formally inform IBL facilitators of the change

2   Develop adequate IT skills to facilitate easy access to resources and information:

- Facilitator IT skills development
- Student IT skills development
- Access to WebCT and additional facilities
- Audit students and staff IT skills competence

3   Provide ongoing support including resources and facilities to enhance the change and encourage a smooth transition:

- Develop Web pages
- Provide documentation in hard copy
- Provide IT resources

Figure 11.1 Modified strategy for implementing the move from paper- to electronic-based information

personal interaction with one another. Indeed, it was expected that students would enjoy the same degree of socialization as they would in an IBL tutorial session.

For the time being the paper-based information system will continue to be run in parallel with the electronic-based one. This is partly a strategy for reducing risk: if there is a catastrophic failure of computer hardware or software, the paper-based system is still in place to provide a fallback position. Also, it remains possible for anyone seeking reassurance about whether the quality of information has been preserved to compare the original paper output with the new computer output. Then too it takes some people longer than others to make the transition to a different way of working, and dual running gives them a little extra time. Of course, there are no cost savings until the paper-based information system is switched off. After the cutoff, everyone will be dependent, in most cases, on the computer for information – although it will continue to be possible to download electronic documents for printing in hard copy when this is a more effective format for working on the material, or as a personal preference.

Web Course Tools (WebCT)

WebCT – which was installed for use by the pre-registration nursing programme at APU in April 2000 – 'enables the institution-wide delivery of online education ... (and) offers a comprehensive solution to meet the needs of the entire educational enterprise' (WebCT 2002). This package was selected because of its functionality, flexibility and customizability. The latter meant that it was possible to switch individual tools and features on or off as needed. Students and staff log on to the system via APU's homepage – either on or off campus using an Internet browser. Each IBL group has its own website (see Figure 11.2).

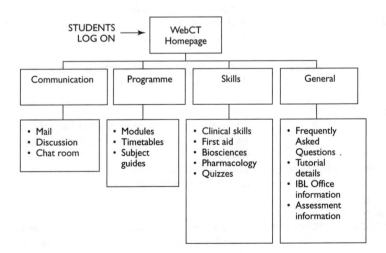

Figure 11.2 WebCT design for IBL students

WebCT features

The WebCT features are summarized in Figure 11.3. There is a variety of student-to-student and student-to-facilitator communication links:

- Chat room: as its name suggests, this is a very informal and immediate mode of communication especially suited to small group work. Remarks and comments are keyed in by each participant to appear, realtime, in the chat that scrolls constantly down the screen. As in live chat, several conversations may be going on at the same time so the various 'threads' become interwoven in the scrolled remarks. As people 'enter' the chat room their screen name is added to the list, displayed on screen, of those already there. When they leave the

TYPE OF FEATURE	PURPOSE
1 COMMUNICATION LINKS	
• **Chat room**	Students can chat online to each other about the programme content
• **Email**	Students can send private messages to their facilitator or to other students
• **Discussion board**	A forum that allows communication among all IBL students
2 PROGRAMME LINKS	
• **Module information**	Students are provided with detailed information about each module
• **Module database**	Students can search for linkable information to complement module content
• **Glossary of terms**	Students are offered the contents as a reference tool.
• **Student presentation** presentations	Students have opportunities for individual and/or group
• **Student self-evaluation**	Students are provided with opportunities to monitor their individual performance
3 SKILLS LINKS	
• **Skills webpage**	This is a resource that helps students learn about bioscience, first aid, pharmacology, psychology, clinical skills, etc.
• **Quiz section**	There is a quiz section for students to test their knowledge of the relevant topics
4 GENERAL INFORMATION LINKS	Students are provided with a variety of programme related information.

Figure 11.3 WebCT features

chat room their screen name is removed from the list. Each IBL group has its own chat room, but students also have access to a chat room dedicated for use by their peer group – all the students that joined in the same year intake. The immediacy of communication in the chat room makes for stimulating exchanges. The main drawback is that, unlike the discussion board, there must be enough people present at the same time to initiate and sustain quick-fire conversation.

- Email tool: an email facility that enables one-to-one messaging – optionally with files attached. Unlike the chat room or the discussion board, this mode of communication is entirely private – although the rest of the group can be copied, which is a useful way to distribute an attached document file. The mail tool allows a student and facilitator to initiate a secure interchange about tutorial or personal issues, or deal with concerns in their entirety if the matter is not serious.

- Discussion board: students can post a message on a topic of interest to the group. The original posting may start a 'thread' of responses from other students that develop the topic further. Some postings attract a lot of interest and most of the group may join in. Others may have a more limited appeal and there might only be two students contributing to the thread. Some topics are of perennial interest and run and run, whilst the content of others is quickly exhausted and the thread peters out. The particular advantage of this asynchronous mode of communication is that participants have time in which to reflect on what has already been posted and to formulate a considered response. Mediated by time as well as the computer, this is a much less anxiety-creating human exchange than face-to-face conversation, and it encourages the sharing of experience that Knowles (1990) thought characteristic of androgogic learning. Because the discussion board allows any number of students to maintain a coherent discussion and they can make their contributions in odd moments outside their scheduled programme activities, Clark (2001) judged it the most flexible of the WebCT tools.

In the programme links, there is information for students about each module in each semester of the IBL programme – including module guides, subject guides, specific module skills laboratory information.

The skills links comprise a number of different topic areas, each of which has its own webpages, PDF (Portable Document Format) documents, PowerPoint presentations and Word documents:

- Skills section: learning resources for bioscience, first aid, pharmacology, psychology, clinical skills, etc.
- Quiz section: students can test their knowledge of a topic by answering questions set by the module leader. Their responses are graded automatically and instantly fed back to the student.

The general information links enable students to access information on, for example, portfolio, frequently asked questions, assessment information, IBL office details, tutorial details, etc.

WebCT tracking

In traditional educational approaches, several aspects of student behaviour – absences, sickness, lateness, non-attendance, for example – are monitored and assessed. Aberrant behaviour that may adversely affect a student's learning is usually considered to be indicative that some form of counselling may be helpful. This simple procedure of collecting and feeding back data so that an appropriate response to any problems identified can be made has been transformed by the introduction of computers. WebCT vastly increases the opportunities for tracking student learning activities – whilst at the same time the cost of data gathering and analysis is reduced to negligible proportions. However, the technology is so powerful and pervasive that, all unawares, it is easy to cross the line that separates watchfulness for the students from surveillance of the students.

One has to tread carefully in this area because there are issues of privacy, confidentiality and ethics to be considered. Students must be told what information is being collected and to what purpose – and educators for their part should ensure that nothing is processed that is to the students' disadvantage. Another important consideration is that there is a level of monitoring that is acceptable to, even welcomed by, the student – because it is understood it has been put in place to deal with that minority of students who do not participate nor make a contribution. If monitoring is increased above that level – so students start to feel they are not trusted – then there is bound to be a deleterious effect on student morale and motivation: most particularly for students in an IBL curriculum. It would be entirely contradictory to expect students to be responsible for their own learning whilst simultaneously demonstrating that the programme's managers have no confidence in the students' ability to behave responsibly.

However, gathering individual statistics like time spent on the system, date of last access, percentage of pages visited, is not likely to be controversial – since these are analogous to the data captured in a traditional register. Nor can there be any objection when data is combined and summarized so individual identity is stripped off. Consolidated information about the numbers and percentages of students accessing each module page is potentially very valuable feedback to programme developers. The feedback reports on student usage of WebCT are sent to the IBL coordinator every three months.

Student and staff development strategy

It is no longer sufficient in contemporary education for students and educators to be merely acquainted with the computer. They must be so familiar and proficient with computing that the interface becomes totally transparent to them in use. They should be no more aware of hardware, software and information processing skills when interacting with electronic information, than they would be of pencil and paper technology and their ability to read and write when making notes from books. One way to encourage and enable that desirable level of unconsciously automatic expertise is to integrate the learning of IT skills into the curriculum – as Bayley *et al.* (2001: 106) advise.

At APU we have done just that for students by introducing an information literacy programme into the pre-registration nursing IBL programme as a fully integrated curriculum strand. In each semester, there is a range of strategies available that enables the steady progression of students and staff from basic to advanced levels of knowledge and practice in information management. The approaches include WebCT training and support packages and, more specifically to the acquisition of generic IT skills, the European Computer Driving Licence (ECDL) – a hands-on instruction programme.

Before students even come to the pre-registration nursing programme at APU they are asked to complete a declaration that they are able to carry out a core repertoire of computer-assisted activities which include word processing, Web search and emails, and that they are able to perform elementary computer operations such as printing and taking backups. The, nowadays fairly rare, potential student who has none of these skills – or more often who has skills acquired in an *ad hoc* fashion that need to be formalized – is encouraged to enrol in an appropriate local adult education course. Once they are on campus and registered for the ECDL programme they have to demonstrate that they actually possess the basic capabilities needed to operate computerized systems: and for this purpose they sit an online test.

The role of the educator

Computerization is the great example in our times of cultural change that alters the way we think and act. In the Western world at least, the generation that is coming into schools of nursing currently is mostly oblivious to this massive paradigm shift – because how things are now is the only reality they have ever experienced. They may not be conversant with the specific architecture and geography of the computer milieu they come into at APU, but they are usually comfortable and 'at home' in it. By contrast, those of their educators from earlier generations are still in the throes of adapting to the novelty of a working environment in which information is becoming predominantly electronically based – with the computer as the sole method of access. (Admittedly, there will be a substantial proportion of the many mature students who will be on that same steep learning curve.)

The logic of the demographics means that, in some aspects of information management, a significant number of students will have a level of knowledge and skill that may well equal or exceed that of their educator. A situation that would result in something of a fiasco in a traditional teacher-centred classroom – since that whole teaching/learning strategy is predicated on the educator being the content expert. The role of the educator in WebCT is exactly the same as it is in any other domain of knowledge in the IBL curriculum. The role of the IBL facilitator is to be a supporter and guide for students in their learning activities: to be, as Alberts (2001) suggests, a mentor, that is, one who is a faithful monitor and wise counsellor.

Student support

It is possible to gain the bare rudiments of information management fairly rapidly and with relatively little effort. Beyond that initial achievement, however, yawns an enormous gulf between those who have just enough IT skills to scrape by, and those who are truly adept – a gulf that can only be spanned by the expenditure of a great deal of time and effort. Even those who have logged many hours of experience with computers already will be ignorant of some areas of the APU systems. The three-stage student support strategy at APU is designed to meet the needs of new students, whether they are relative novices or experts, and the needs of existing students who started their programme with a mostly paper-based information system and must make the transition to a largely electronically based system. Since students are self-directed and have their own individual educational requirements, the three stages of the strategy may be expanded, compressed or conflated to suit individual requirements.

The first stage of the student support strategy is developing awareness. At APU, students are provided with information about what the computer literacy expectations are, how to assess their skill attainments, where to find programme documents on WebCT and details about hardware/software. The existing students in transition from paper- to electronic-based information were kept informed on progress by feedback from their representatives at planning meetings, with online and on-board notices, and, as implementation approached, by personal letter to each individual student.

The second stage is orientation to the use of information technology at APU. Students, whether new or transitional, need to be kept informed of the particular mix of hardware, software and netware that they will be expected to interface with – as it is updated, replaced and expanded to provide new services and functionality. This is accomplished by posting orientation information, with a help page, on the Web and holding orientation sessions. Whilst much of this orientation is intellectual an important element is attitudinal. It is no coincidence that the students who benefit most from electronically based information systems are those who benefit most from the IBL approach. They are the self-directed learners who work equally well independently or networking with the group. Students are encouraged to reflect on their own attitudes to information technology and its place in relating to others as part of their overall orientation.

The third stage is ongoing technology support. Technical help is most intensive when new users are logging on WebCT and other online services within APU and externally on the Internet. In the first few weeks it functions effectively as the knowledge resource of last resort during orientation when students are finding their way with unfamiliar hardware, software and netware. Technical help is a constant thereafter where it is called upon for advice on the more esoteric components of the system, or to deal with operational malfunction – the bugbear of all complex IT structures.

Local and central technical support for students, and others, comes from APU computer and information services and health schools sited IT trainer and technicians. Support is delivered by telephone, email, consultation and training sessions.

Staff support

Just like students, staff also need to be supported with awareness briefings, orientation sessions in the hardware, software and netware and ongoing technical help – and the time to acquire the requisite knowledge and skills. The natural affinity between student-directed learning and electronically sourced information has already been mentioned – it is an example of the perfect match of man and machine. Part of the role of the IBL facilitator in that relationship is to develop learning materials for uploading to WebCT and other systems for access by the IBL students. This task involves the deployment of specialist information management skills which require a specific programme of planned staff development.

Conclusion

Implementing WebCT, moving from paper-based to mainly electronic-based information, is revolutionary. And it has taken place in an educational environment that is itself undergoing revolutionary change. Fortunately, the changes are mutually supportive, with the profile of the ideal IBL student – independent, self-directed, questioning – matching the profile of the ideal WebCT user.

Chapter 12

Subproject 7: library resources

Introduction

Making a difference (Department of Health 1999), the Government strategy to raise standards in nursing, midwifery and health visiting called for, amongst other things, a more flexible approach to the education of nurses – for example, the implementation of problem-based and enquiry-based learning as possible ways forward. This in turn prompted the University Health Sciences Librarians (2001) to develop a strategy for the support of, and resource provision for, any such new direction in nurse education by library and information services. Since student-centred learning is, by definition, diametrically opposed to teacher-centred learning it follows that the optimal library service for each will also be very different.

A library set up to serve students in a teacher-centred approach is able to plan its provision with a high degree of certainty. It is likely to know well in advance the set course texts and suggested further reading, and the number of students who are going to be borrowing or referencing each of these texts. For the teacher-directed student, the university library is not a store of all human knowledge – just the place they keep the set books in.

The library that has to cater for the student-centred approach has to plan the services it offers and the resources it provides on the basis of probabilities, not certainties. The IBL students in the exploration tutorial work through a scenario together, generating learning issues as they go. As part of their self-directed explorations the students will access a range of resources, one of which is invariably the library. But IBL students arrive at the library in ones and twos, perhaps a whole IBL group, with a list of questions and unresolved learning issues, not a list of the books which they have been instructed to read. It is the teacher-centred learners who assume they know which books the answers are in before they even get to the library – their behaviour is essentially deterministic. The IBL student is obliged to perform a wide-ranging search for answers: browsing the shelves, accessing many classifications, tracking down primary sources – and, since active learners are encouraged to be intellectually curious, now and then reading slightly, sometimes completely, off topic.

The IBL students may not necessarily know in advance what library resources their search for answers will range across – but because they are many and their behaviour is random it is susceptible to statistical analysis to estimate likely usages. Post-implementation, as patterns of actual use begin to emerge, the librarian may be able to estimate the probable demands of IBL students for core materials with improved accuracy, and purchase stock accordingly. However, for much, perhaps most, of the range of materials held by the library, the individual usage frequencies will be too low to give statistical authority to decisions about retaining or discontinuing particular items and these will remain a matter for the judgement of librarians and their academic colleagues. In any event, the library needs to offer an exceptionally broad choice of materials because the student-directed learner forages over such a wide range of material. This active, extensive, exploratory pattern of usage appears to be the case at APU where the IBL students seem to be making relatively heavy demands on library resources, according to Wakeham (2000), the subject librarian for nursing.

There is a great deal of corroborating evidence attesting to the distinctive 'library' behaviours of traditional and student-centred learners and the characteristically more active library usage of the latter (see Figure 12.1).

TRADITIONAL STUDENTS	STUDENT-CENTRED STUDENTS (PBL)	COMMENTATOR
Lesser library use	Greater library use	Rankin (1992)
Use less resources material	Use more resources material	Blumberg and Michael (1992)
Use library less	Use library: • More frequently • With longer visits	Marshall et al. (1993)
Less extensive use of print material	Extensive use of print material	Blake (1994)
Use library less often	Use library more often	
Libraries and information services used less	Libraries and information services used more	Rankin (1996)
Use library later and less often	Use library earlier and more often	Bechtel et al. (1999)

Figure 12.1 Traditional and student-centred students' library behaviours

The research evidence noted above was taken into the decision-making process in the early planning stages of implementing the IBL curriculum. The importance of adequate library provision to the success of the project cannot be overemphasized

– as the Jackson and Parker (1998: 175) list of the crucial services a library offers to students makes clear:

- provision of resources for learning and teaching
- access to these resources
- skills teaching for the learner
- provision of ongoing advice, guidance and support.

Provision of resources

Because the demands that student-directed learners make on a library are so very different both in kind and in degree from those that can be expected of students working in more traditional curricula, librarians must be included at the heart, and at the start, of the implementation process. Late involvement can be the cause of much frustration to those responsible for library services, as reported by University Health Sciences Librarians (2001), quite apart from missing an opportunity to eliminate an avoidable risk to project success. At APU, the librarian was involved formally and informally at an early stage in the IBL curriculum planning and development: serving on the curriculum and field committees as a resource person so as to be 'aware of the precise information needs of the course of study before the course begins so that appropriate resources may be acquired and the skills to use these resources transmitted' (Jackson and Parker 1998: 176).

An awareness session for the library staff at the university and in the NHS trust libraries that supported pre-registration nursing students was given by the IBL coordinator in liaison with the subject librarian to reorient them to the different needs of IBL students. A wide selection of off-line resources are available to support learning. As might be expected books, journals and other printed material form a significant part of this provision. Photocopiers can be accessed with smart cards by students. Additionally, the library buys in commercial videos for viewing locally. Librarians also, in collaboration with media production, make copies of broadcast programmes, under licence. This might be at the instigation of academic staff members but very often is on the librarians' own initiative.

Computer workstations are installed in the library for students to access the constantly expanding universe of online material – an IT resource that is separate from and additional to the computers that each IBL group has in their own 'home base' IBL room. The university library website's health and nursing resources pages include:

- subject topics
- subject gateways to, for example, National Electronic Library for Health
- databases, such as the BNI (British Nursing Index), CINAHL (Cumulative Index in Nursing and Allied Health Literature)
- organizations such as Department of Health
- electronic journals.

Access to resources

Because IBL students use the library more often, and stay in the library for longer periods when they do, the access facilities they require involve far more than the simple procedures for borrowing and returning books that are characteristic of library use in traditional pedagogy. The primary necessity as far as access is concerned is that the library should be open. At APU, the library is typically open from 8.30 a.m. to midnight – allowing long, uninterrupted periods of study to be sustained as well as accommodating the variety in individual demand that is implicit in learning that is self-directed.

As Jackson and Parker (1998) indicate, a suitable place in which to study that gives ready access to materials is a prerequisite for learning. In the IBL context, that includes not just the individual student working alone, but also small groups of students working together. The library provides group study rooms for this purpose. The use of the library as a place to meet other students was remarked upon by Marshall *et al.* (1993) – speaking of PBL students, but the same behaviour can be observed with the IBL students at APU. It is an opportunity to make arrangements with other group members to study together at scheduled non-facilitated times as well as a chance to share experiences with students from other groups.

Library skills development

Some basic library skills are intuitive, or were acquired so long ago in childhood they might as well be considered so. But the extensive range of material and the diversity of the technology needed to access it means that all students will benefit from an enhancement and extension of their library skills, as Walton and Matthews (1989) discovered. The library skills orientation and development programme at APU is coordinated by the subject librarian.

In an introductory tour, on day two of their first week at APU, students newly enrolled on the pre-registration nursing programme are taken around the library – usually in their IBL groups. The purpose of the tour is to welcome the students and give a general orientation. They meet and learn the names of the staff who will be assisting them. Each student is given a 'Guide for Students' booklet and shown the basic services and layout, procedures and the off-line resources, including:

- where and how to borrow books
- self-issue procedure
- fines
- journals
- photocopiers, audio-visual equipment and workstations
- group study and training rooms.

During their first four weeks students take part in scheduled sessions in the library training room, in which they are introduced to the online library catalogue and website. In hands-on mode they learn how to use the catalogue to find and reserve books and renew loans. They also learn how to access online resources, especially the health and nursing webpages.

Ongoing support

Drop-in sessions cater to small IBL groups and individuals who need a one-to-one level of assistance – perhaps mature techno-phobic students who need encouragement, or other students who lack confidence or who have fallen behind their peers for some other reason. Additional or alternative options, which also address the needs of students who are unable to attend the usual sessions, are the standard library skills programme provided by APU, and the self-help materials – online or print – produced by library staff.

A variety of other ongoing support and guidance is available. There are online and print resource guides and access to help-lines via telephone, email or online. The collaboration between the APU health schools and the local NHS trusts and Workforce Development Confederation, described by Wakeham (2000), ensures that IBL students on placement in the pre-registration nursing programme can be similarly supported by local NHS libraries.

Conclusion

The implementation and onward progress of the IBL curriculum has revolutionized the learning process in the pre-registration nursing programme at APU. The staff of the university and NHS libraries have responded to this different and larger demand by rapidly evolving new resources and services and expanding the capacity of existing ones. It is no surprise that they been able to help and support IBL students so effectively – after all, encouraging and facilitating the learning activities of others has always been an important attribute of the librarian's role.

Chapter 13

Subproject 8: media resources

Introduction

Operationalizing the whole IBL curriculum necessarily involves managing a vast array of information using many different media. This chapter focuses on that subset of the technological infrastructure that enables speech and/or images to be stored permanently or temporarily for later retrieval – the audio-visual aids (AVA). Print and computer resources are examined elsewhere. The AVAs available to the IBL students in the pre-registration nursing programme include:

- digital camera
- overhead projector
- tele-video
- video camera
- flipchart
- whiteboard
- audio-cassette recorder.

None of these devices would be out of place in a traditional classroom. The progressive educator must therefore bear in mind that AVAs have the potential to induce passivity and care has to be taken to use them only in ways that call for active participative learning by students.

The spoken word is not the most effective method of communicating new concepts or information that goes much beyond what is already understood. Nevertheless, Confucius's famous hierarchy of memorability is perhaps too absolute in its terms, 'I hear and I forget, I see and I remember, I do and I understand'. One has only to consider how quickly and efficiently a joke is transmitted to appreciate that oral communication can be effective. We think a joke funny when it surprises us with a truth about our own lives – and the shock of the insight fixes it in memory. We are stimulated, we actively participate, we remember. But the content of lengthy speech cannot be retained so easily – even the greatest orators are remembered for a few telling phrases; everything else is forgotten.

Edgar Dale's 'cone of learning' proposes that two weeks after learning people remember:

10 percent of what they read
20 percent of what they hear
30 percent of what they see
50 percent of what they see and hear
70 percent of what they say
90 percent of what they both say and do

(cited by Integrated Technologies, Inc. 2002)

It follows from this model that the use of AVA will tend to increase retention by including the two senses of hearing and seeing simultaneously. But, at their best, AVAs may be able to improve on that and bring more of Dale's triad of hear, see and do, into play by engaging the imaginations of students to such an extent that they enjoy a virtual learning experience – in effect they 'do' by acting out in their imaginations as well as 'see' and 'hear'. In spite of that, it should not be forgotten that AVAs are more typically tools of passive learning and, as such, need to be treated with a good deal of caution, especially when used in a curriculum that depends on active learning for its success. However, AVAs can extend the range and quality of learning experiences, and in an IBL context, this is of especial value because it gives the self-directed learner more scope to choose specific learning experiences that will contribute whatever is most needed in the construction of the learner's own individual knowledge base and skills.

Purpose of AVAs

The purpose of AVAs is to provide secondary support to the learning process. These mechanical aids achieve this purpose in three ways:

- by providing sources of supplementary information
- by giving learners access to material that they would not otherwise be able to obtain
- by conveying information that cannot be communicated as effectively in any other way.

In the traditional classroom, the use of an AVA was very often no more than a tactic to continue the lecture by other means, i.e. as a surrogate for the teacher. In an IBL environment, an AVA should never be more than ancillary to the tutorial learning process. That process relies for its educational effect on human interaction in a small group and would be swiftly derailed if an AVA moved to centre stage. The purpose of an AVA is to give the supplementary information that rounds out what has been learned and puts it into context, to contribute those telling details and concrete examples that help to make the abstract concepts developed in the tutorial process memorable. If the module scenario is based on care of the elderly then the group's explorations will not be assisted by a training video on care of the elderly that repeats the knowledge the group has already developed for itself – but a video of pensioners reminiscing may well throw a new light on what has been learned and bring new understanding.

A second purpose of AVAs is to convey information that cannot be easily accessed in any other way, e.g. a voyage through the gastrointestinal tract by endoscope. There is a multitude of objects and events that are too small or too large, too fast or too slow, too infrequent, too dangerous and so on, to be observed by the human senses without the mediation of some sort of AVA. In spite of its intrinsic interest, such material should still only be used when it is germane to the topics being explored in the IBL tutorial process. Otherwise the IBL group may lose focus or be encouraged to venture down unproductive avenues.

Lastly, there are times when an AVA is the medium of choice. All the AVAs that have blank media which can be used by students to record their comments and conclusions fall into this category, e.g. flipchart, whiteboard, audio recorder, video camera. These devices allow two-way communication – write and read, record and play – and are therefore aids to active learning. Indeed the small IBL group in tutorial session exemplifies active learning, and flipchart and whiteboard are both integral components of that learning process.

In the traditional classroom an important purpose of AVAs was to revive students whose normal passivity had degenerated into downright boredom as a consequence of listening to overlong expositions from their teacher. In the teacher-directed mode of instruction, a condition of relative lack of learning responsiveness generally sets in about every fifteen to twenty minutes. This state of learning resistance has been diagnosed as due to 'information overload' or 'mental fatigue', though these terms suggest students have learned too much, too rapidly – which seems improbable given the students' inactivity and lack of involvement. In IBL the students are self-directed, active and involved. If the group loses motivation in a session then it should be able to find a more interesting and productive learning activity by itself. It is quite likely that the IBL facilitator might suggest at such a juncture using an AVA as a way of helping the group to identify a new area for exploration. There is no place in IBL for using AVAs as a palliative to recurrent boredom – if a particular student is bored then, after reflection, the facilitator will intervene correctively at an individual level. It is only the teacher-directed students who need to be refreshed continually so they can return to more of the same – the IBL group simply chooses to do something different.

Types of AVA

There is a wide variety of AVAs available for IBL student use at APU: ranging from simple tools to state of the art electronic kit. The assortment of AVA devices that are standard fittings in each of the IBL rooms is discussed briefly below.

- Flipcharts and whiteboards: these are indispensable props in the tutorial process, as has been mentioned already. The IBL group scribe records the points made in the IBL session, as they are raised, on the flipchart – where what is being written remains on view for instant verification. Rough hand-written notes are best for this work because it is easy to cross out or amend comments as the group's thinking evolves, or to reinstate discarded items which on reflection need to be included. In the exploration tutorial, the flipchart or whiteboard is used to jot down the ideas generated during brainstorming sessions. A more formal use is in the review tutorial, as display aids in student presentations of what they have discovered in their self-directed learning time – for which flipchart pages may be prepared in advance.
- Overhead projectors (OHP), slide projectors and PowerPoint: these are conceptually very similar although the last of these is a much more expressive medium than the first two. All are easy to use, versatile, and for these reasons, popular visual aids. Text and images can be transferred to transparencies/slides/ frames in advance of the presentation, and reveals and overlays used during presentation – making it possible to display ideas in a logical and entertaining manner.
- Videotape recorders and camcorders: these can be used in a conventional way to show commercial, library or media production sourced documentary material. Of greater interest and value educationally is the use by students of camcorders: to capture material that is of special relevance to them – in effect shooting their own documentaries; or to make a filmed record of an individual review presentation for subsequent critical assessment with the whole IBL group and facilitator – feeding back improvements into future performances.
- Audiotape: this is by no means a poor relation of more sophisticated tech-nologies. It is inexpensive, simple to use and unobtrusive – therefore eminently suited to the needs of the lone operator recording social interactions. As a medium, sound recording is noted for its capacity to communicate descriptions by individuals of their personal thoughts and feelings with a great deal of psychological realism and emotional force.

Student support

In the contemporary educational scene, the media technologies are no longer an external function, like catering or estates, that may provide a valuable service to the teaching and learning process but are not an integral part of it. At APU, the media production department is still responsible as always for producing print and other materials, for providing, maintaining and sometimes operating equipment, stocking consumables, and so on, but additionally and importantly, it also has a direct role in helping students to acquire a wide range of media skills, most especially in the use of AVA resources which include, but are not limited to, technical instruction. Working with the media resources staff, the students also gain the higher order knowledge of design, authoring, editing and publishing. These have become core skills now that so much essential information is held electronically – acquiring them brings an immediate payoff in the students' academic lives, and in future will continue to benefit them in their professional careers and in lifelong learning.

Conclusion

Media production, often working in concert with the librarians and academics, seeks 'to provide a complete audiovisual media . . . service' (Harris 1996: 196). The high profile of AVAs in the IBL curriculum – a prominence that has become more emphatic with the move away from paper-based and towards electronic-based information – has made the acquisition of media skills by students an educational priority.

AVAs play a vital role in the delivery of the IBL pre-registration nursing programme. Although they make a unique contribution, it is one that should be used with discretion and focus. The heavy and enthusiastic reliance on AVAs in teacher-centred approaches – as a periodic spur when student attention flags – is a warning that their indiscriminate use in IBL can undermine active learning by substituting ready answers for self-directed lines of inquiry.

Part IV

By the time tomorrow comes

Chapter 14

Where are we now?

Introduction

At APU we have achieved so much of which to be proud that it is difficult to accept that we are still only in the early stages of implementing the whole IBL curriculum. Indeed, we should not claim to have achieved much more than survival. Admittedly, the quality of our initial planning and development decisions and actions has been tested now in the fire of live operation and has not been found wanting. But it is apparent that much remains to be done and that planners and developers must regroup to prepare themselves – and the many others involved in delivering and using the IBL pre-registration nursing programme – for the move forward into the next stage of the IBL curriculum's development. For move forward we must, or we stand to lose everything we have gained so far. The enemies of progress – fear, sloth, apathy and pessimism – though we reduce them to shadows of their former selves by managing change effectively, never fade away entirely and whilst it is still in its infancy the IBL project remains especially vulnerable to such negative impulses. So, paradoxically, the safest way to defend what we have already achieved is to move forward, to keep up the rate of change, to maintain momentum.

It was the leadership and vision of the APU health schools, the Workforce Development Confederation and the local NHS trusts, all working together in partnership, that overcame the initial inertia and got the IBL project up and running. And it is the continued support and guidance of these bodies over the first two years that has kept the IBL implementation up to speed and pointed in the right direction. If there is a single key factor, one thing that made the project a success rather than a failure, it was the high level of involvement. Being an onlooker, a bystander or any sort of non-participant were not acceptable options. Involvement – meaning taking responsibility, consultation, concern, cooperation, commitment, contribution – of students, academics, practitioners and support staff was the constant priority that influenced every decision and shaped every action.

IBL is a model of learning whose time has come. All kinds of educational institutions in many parts of the world are searching for a way to break through the glass ceiling that teacher-directed strategies impose on learning. They want to push past the old limitations and release the full potential of their students and staff – and they are looking to inquiry-based or problem-based approaches to learning to do this for them. Many of these institutions have elected to trial PBL in selected learning modules, units or short courses. On the surface this seems to promise the attractive prospect of a low cost, low risk transition from teacher-directed to student-directed learning. A stumbling block may be the unfortunate students who are expected to behave with consistency and authenticity in two completely opposing ways – either directing/being directed, or active/passive, or talking/listening, or asking/being told – switching persona according to what sort of session they find themselves in. It is difficult to see what valid conclusions can be gained from such a bewildering exercise.

Process of momentum

Once a project's momentum is lost, the novelty soon wears off, management attention switches away to focus on the next big thing, general enthusiasm fizzles out as staff realize that what had been so enjoyable to do in staff development is not nearly so much fun in day to day practice. As enthusiasm drains away, the backsliding begins. The enemies of progress renew their attacks: the philosophy is tuned in the name of so-called 'commonsense', the methodology is tinkered with to make it fit 'tried and true' recipes – and very soon everything that is new or different has been unravelled or corrupted. The operation reverts to its previous, pre-implementation, state. It may still look as if a great change has taken place – the new titles, new equipment, redecorations, etc. are still much in evidence – but underneath surface appearances, change has died and the old system has quietly re-established itself.

Naturally we were anxious to avoid this all too common scenario. We knew that the momentum that we had built up with such effort, and to such effect, in the development phase of the IBL curriculum project had to be maintained after implementation – to fend off any reactionary tendencies seeking to halt and reverse the changes we wanted to make. Accordingly, the strategic and operational management infrastructure has been retained – including the IBL coordinator. The IBL community is kept up to date with news and developments, and, importantly, IBL specific staff development, for academics and practitioners to enhance skills and reinforce commitment, continues apace.

Unfortunately, as Miller (1990) revealed, the good thing about momentum – that it helps to keep the operation running exactly the way the planners and developers intended it should – is also the bad thing – it makes it hard to change direction. In a changing world, the inability to respond appropriately, or at all, to meet the challenges of new circumstances spells disaster. Maintaining sufficient forward impetus to keep the IBL curriculum project energized and focused, whilst preventing the rigid purpose and blinkered vision of excessive momentum, can be achieved by deciding what the ultimate objective of the curriculum should be, and making as many changes in direction as are needed to keep that destination constantly in sight. The quality concept offers a convenient and credible model of what that objective should be, namely, 'delighting the users' (Peters 1994, cited by Koltay and Calhoun 2002: 1).

Chapter 15

Where are we going?

Introduction

Deciding who the end-users of the pre-registration nursing programme might be is not so straightforward. The student considers the programme's product to be their own education. The service employer considers the programme's product to be a qualified, registered practitioner. The client/patient considers the programme's product to be the nursing care that they receive. Although there is a high degree of overlap in what these very different users want, there is obviously quite a wide spread of programme outcomes to be achieved before we can say that we are delighting each and every one of them. This would be a daunting prospect if we did not have two excellent tools to deal with achieving multiple objectives – namely, the IBL curriculum and quality management.

The IBL curriculum has the capacity to accommodate a variety of outcomes because it does not limit itself to vocational training but provides a whole education. Potentially, the IBL student learns how to learn, learns the knowledge and skills for both caring and sharing – and more besides. The student user should secure that richness of professional and personal skills that makes for confident and able practice. The employer user should get a professional practitioner with advanced learning skills, one who is able to become an even more productive employee in post, by mastering additional competencies and by keeping up with new developments. A professional practitioner who has, moreover, the social skills that optimize team productivity. The patient/client user will enjoy receiving nursing care – in terms of knowledge, skills and attitudes – of a high order.

The quality approach deals with the complexity of multiple outcomes by treating error not as a mistake for which a culprit must be found and punished, but rather as an indicator signifying that desired outcomes are no longer being achieved. Once errors are corrected, the desired outcomes start to be achieved again. This simple technique ensures the operation remains focused on its objectives – if it drifts off target, the increase in errors sounds the alarm; as the errors are corrected, the operation moves back on target. Borrowing heavily from quality models which are in wide use, it should be possible to describe a development path for the IBL curriculum that can take us from where we are now in a series of logical steps to our ultimate objective of 'delighting the users'.

Davies (1991) identified three stages in the evolution of an organization's total quality management system. Suitably customized, using the author's personal knowledge and experience, these became the initial building blocks for a new model of curriculum evolution. With the addition of 'enlightenment' as a final inspirational stage – from Crosby's (1997) Quality Management Maturity Grid – the four-stage model was complete (see Figure 15.1):

1   Endurance
2   Elimination
3   Enhancement
4   Enlightenment.

Although the stages are shown as compartmentalized, they are not really totally exclusive one from another. Just as primitive and advanced traits are present in each individual human, so a particular organization may exhibit elements of behaviour from more than one stage.

Stage 1: Endurance

In the endurance stage the curriculum functions well enough for survival purposes. The implementation team is aware of the key problems, is taking action to correct them and setting up procedures to prevent those errors recurring. The culture is reactive and blaming. Management tends to wait for complaints to reach a high level before taking action. This situation is a common one and most curricula do not evolve beyond it.

Stage 2: Elimination

In the elimination stage the curriculum is periodically reviewed to make it more effective and more efficient. Error detection is a formal exercise directed at elimination and prevention before problems occur. The culture is proactive and values people – staff development is a high priority. The value of quality management in the curriculum is acknowledged – but more in principle than in practice.

Stage 3: Enhancement

This stage is rarely encountered in any type of institution. In education, the enhancement stage would be one in which the curriculum is a completely integrated process in which students, academics, practitioners and support staff work in harmony to achieve its outcomes. The culture is participative and quality is everyone's responsibility.

STAGE 1: ENDURANCE DURATION: 1 to 2 YEARS	STAGE 2: ELIMINATION DURATION: 3 to 5 YEARS	STAGE 3: ENHANCEMENT DURATION: 5 to 7 YEARS	STAGE 4: ENLIGHTENMENT DURATION: 7 or more YEARS
1. Tend to blame others for curriculum problems	7. Bringing the curriculum 'under control'	13. Curriculum is an integrated process	19. Benefiting everyone
2. Problems are fought as they occur	8. Challenging existing roles and methods	14. Total user orientation	20. Strong sense of ownership
3. Recognizing competitive threat and the need for improvement	9. Teams are set up to attack major problems	15. Fully participative management	21. Development of new ideas
4. Isolating key problems	10. Building quality into the curriculum	16. Controlled continuous enhancement is the norm	22. Meaningful communications are established
5. Organizing to solve problems	11. Developing capable and motivated people	17. All staff actively participating in the enhancement process	23. Management committed to quality
6. Solve the problems	12. Defect prevention becomes routine	18. Management becomes more supportive and helpful	24. Commitment to user
			25. Delighting the user

Figure 15.1 Curriculum evolution: the four stages of development

Stage 4: Enlightenment

> With the establishment of a regular quality policy, and the admission that we
> cause our own problems, management enters the stage of Enlightenment.
>
> (Crosby 1979: 34)

This is what we are aiming for – the IBL curriculum as a fully realized quality
process which routinely delights its users. Of course it is not an error free environment – nor can it ever be. The users will always be wanting something new from
the pre-registration nursing programme and the IBL curriculum will be redeveloped
to deliver those new outcomes. Whenever the goalposts are moved in this way,
there are bound to be a few misses whilst the error correcting procedures kick in to
realign everything on the changed objectives.

'Change is a slow and difficult process' (Cole 1996: 92). It takes time to progress
through the four stages of curriculum evolution – a 'guesstimate' of possible
durations, after Davies (1991), is given for each stage shown in Figure 15.1.

Planning for transition

Most institutions are in the endurance stage, though many of these may have some
stage two features. The large-scale organizational change that APU underwent to
implement the IBL curriculum had the effect of moving us up into the elimination
stage of curriculum evolution. It must be confessed, however, that we are guilty
from time to time of displaying stage one behaviours, and there are stage two
behaviours that we have yet to master. Deciding, as exactly as one can, where one
is currently is important if the transition to the next stage is to be made in an orderly
fashion. To help make that assessment, the subprojects of the curriculum infrastructure that we developed to manage the IBL implementation are used as examples
(see Part III). The subprojects are:

- staff development
- communication system
- classroom compass
- practice experience
- documentation
- electronic resources
- library resources
- media resources.

Taking the staff development segment as an example of how a review profile based
on these subprojects might be used: if, faced with a staff problem, a manager
typically thinks 'disciplinary procedures', they are in the endurance stage; if 'staff
development', they are in the elimination stage. It is possible to devise a fairly
detailed quality checklist for the key activities in each of the subprojects. This
exercise should enable a well-founded plan for transition to be developed.

Chapter 16

Postscript

The experience of implementing IBL in the pre-registration nursing curriculum has been an education and a revelation. We learned things we did not know, and finally came to really understand things we thought we already knew. Because we were implementing a whole curriculum we had to review the entire infrastructure. Sometimes we found that not only did it not meet the needs of the new curriculum, it failed to meet all the needs of the existing curriculum. We learned there are huge dividends – in terms of user productivity and satisfaction – to be gained by taking a lot of trouble to tune processes to meet the needs of those using them, instead of relying on the ingenuity and effort of users to make ill-matched systems function. Most importantly, we rediscovered the truth of something we already knew, that the golden dividend comes from investing in people. They are the universal lubricant that makes everything work better – time and money spent on involving and developing staff is time and money well spent.

Undoubtedly, our transition from the endurance to the elimination stage was greatly aided by the fact that a new philosophy and methodology meant we could start over and build the new curriculum without having to accommodate any hostages from the past. Then too the IBL philosophy is highly compatible with total quality management concepts, both being infused with rationalist and humanist ideals so the onward evolution of the curriculum should be a less dramatic and unsettling experience than at the start.

Of one thing we can be utterly certain – by the time tomorrow comes the curriculum will be different – very likely, very different – from the one that we have implemented. Change comes from all directions. Externally: from government and statutory bodies – a recent and major example being multi-professional IBL groups – and from market forces, where the rise and fall of competing educational institutions forces offensive/defensive adaptations to our offerings. Internally and locally: from building quality into the curriculum; to respond to policy and strategy initiatives from university level and our Workforce Development Confederation and NHS trust partners. And, not least, in a self-directed approach students have a big say in curriculum functionality – the 'take it or leave it' attitude of traditional pedagogy will not do at all.

Change will happen. If we do not make the changes ourselves – change happens anyway. So – by the time tomorrow comes – be prepared!

Postgraduate student's reflection: extracts

Facilitating Inquiry-Based Learning module

Reflective diary entry: 'My starting point', 10 January 2002

IBL Residential

My thoughts prior to the residential:

Facilitation . . . yes I can do that. I have a facilitative style of teaching anyway. I'm comfortable with it as a way of teaching and learning. I know we [as a team] may have difficulty because we don't all feel very comfortable with it.

12 January 2002

These three days have been *brilliant!* The actual lived experience of doing IBL from a student's perspective has enabled me to know what it is all about. I needed that experience. It's one thing to have the theory, another thing to put it into practice. I think one of the most important messages I'm taking away is the importance of understanding the IBL process and using *all* steps of the process. Each step must be undertaken if IBL is to be successful. Attendees at this residential . . . who have experienced facilitation of IBL processes . . . identified that problems occurred with the IBL process and the students understanding of their role within it when lecturers were doing something a bit different . . .

It seems to me that what is *crucial* to all this working is to prepare the facilitators *and* placement staff for their roles within the IBL process. Importance of looking at preconceptions of IBL. Motivation levels. People need to be fully committed to the process otherwise they approach it half-heartedly. This may result in students getting mixed messages, confused, learning hindered and the whole process falls down.

There was debate about whether one should be an expert in the subject area, which was interesting, not sure which side of the fence I fall down on yet. Will I be able to stop myself from taking over a discussion on a subject I am passionate about . . . ? It seems facilitators *do* need to have a very good understanding of IBL and facilitation process. In fact it can hinder the process because you would be more likely to step in and take over or answer the question for the students. This gives mixed messages and confuses students and hinders learning.

Virtual IBL group: Extract from workbook

Postgraduate Module: facilitating Inquiry-Based Learning

Virtual Inquiry-Based Learning Group

(Based on a storyboard approach)

The Virtual Inquiry-Based Learning (IBL) Group is designed as a support and enhancement of experience gained in live IBL groups and for the empowerment of module participants. In the module, a storyboard performs the function of interface between participants and a virtual IBL student group.

First, the approach will stimulate and challenge participants to advance their attitudes, skills and knowledge of working with small groups of students. Second, it will assist participants to address the related scenario issues and module outcomes. Lastly, the use of the storyboard/virtual group is a practical demonstration of IBL's capacity to utilize novel learning methods as a stimulus to learning – in addition to a wide variety of conventional techniques.

Outline

Virtual group	Eight students and a facilitator. The group seems to be well balanced and heterogeneous. Minority students are represented. No identified type of student is concentrated in the group.
Context	Inquiry-Based Learning tutorial
Venue	Inquiry-Based Learning room
Key players	Facilitator and students

Students			
	1	Mandy	Very shy. Her whispers could hardly be heard.
	2	Bumi	Has been in this country only a few weeks. She is clearly uncomfortable speaking in public.
	3	Stephen	Enjoys the limelight and is very out-spoken.
	4	Gail	Very bright, but unreliable.
	5	Ayo	An extrovert, she is less committed to the group.
	6	Ann-Marie	Conscientious, pleasant and contributes well to the group.
	7	Linda	Keen, committed to the group.
	8	Emma	Enthusiastic and sociable.

Participants will be required to undertake the Virtual IBL Group exercises during self-directed learning – unscheduled time, individually or with others.

Participants will be encouraged to work from webpages which can only be accessed by using a password.

Storyboard scenario titles
Absenteeism and lateness

Core concepts
- Attendance
- Punctuality
- Participation
- Cooperative learning
- Conflicts
- Group dynamics

Images and Captions: See individual storyboard.

Exercise: Based on the IBL tutorial process.

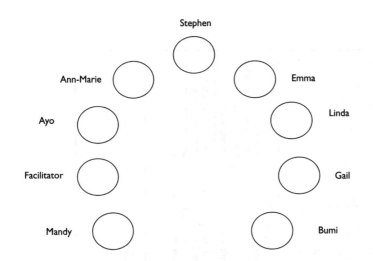

Figure A2.1 Virtual IBL group – room plan

Exercise: Apply the IBL tutorial process to the scenario

Scenario title: Absenteeism and lateness

Gail regularly misses one IBL tutorial in each module.

Emma has missed four IBL tutorials this module – due to a fractured femur.

Ayo is late for tutorials as usual.

The remaining students resent Gail and Ayo because they disrupt the activities of the group.

Linda asked you whether it is possible to drop someone from the group.

- What could you have done to avoid these problems?
- What should you do now?

Core concepts

Attendance
Punctuality
Participation
Cooperative learning
Conflicts
Group dynamics

Scenario title: Absenteeism and lateness

Images				
Set	Seven students and the facilitator sit in a semi-circle. 1 empty seat	Six students and the facilitator sit in a semi-circle. 2 empty seats	Five students and the facilitator sit in a semi-circle. 3 empty seats	Six students and the facilitator sit in a semi-circle. 2 empty seats	Six students and the facilitator sit in a semi-circle. One student talks to the facilitator. 2 empty seats
Caption	Gail regularly misses one IBL tutorial in each module.	Emma has missed four IBL tutorials this module – due to a fractured femur.	Ayo is late for tutorials, as usual.	The remaining students resent Gail and Ayo because they disrupt the activities of the group.	Linda asks facilitator if it is possible to drop someone from the group.

Additional exercise: What could you have done to avoid these problems? What should you do now?

Key	● Missing student	● Late arrival	● Facilitator	○ F

Figure A2.2 Storyboard exercise 1: Apply the IBL tutorial process to the scenario

References

Alavi, C. (1995) *Problem-Based Learning in a Health Sciences Curriculum*. London: Routledge.

Alavi, C. and Cook, M. (1995) Assessing Problem-Based Learning, in C. Alavi (ed.), *Problem-Based Learning in a Health Sciences Curriculum*. London: Routledge.

Alberts, P.P. (2001) Instructional Design: Skills Required by Lecturers in WebCT Based Courses, in the Third Annual WebCT Conference: Transforming the Educational Experience. Vancouver, B.C., Canada: June 23–27, 2001.

Allen, D.E., Duch, B.J. and Groh, S.E. (2001) Strategies for Using Groups, in B.J. Duch, S.E. Groh and D.E. Allen (eds), *The Power of Problem-Based Learning*. Virginia: Stylus Publishing.

Anderson, B. (1992) Task and Reflection in Learning to Learn, in J. Mulligan and C. Griffin (eds), *Empowerment through Experiential Learning*. London: Kogan Page Ltd.

Andrews, J. (1995) Effective Communication, in D. Warner and E. Crosthwaite (eds), *Human Resource Management in Higher and Further Education*. Buckingham: SRHE and Open University Press.

Apps, J. (1985) *Improving Practice in Continuing Education*. London: Jossey-Bass Inc.

Apps, J. (1988) *Higher Education in a Learning Society*. London: Jossey-Bass Inc.

Ballantyne, R., Borthwick, J. and Packer, J. (2000) Beyond Student Evaluation of Teaching: Identifying and Addressing Academic Staff Development Needs. *Assessment and Evaluation in Higher Education*, 25 (3): 221–236.

Barrows, H.S. (1986) A Taxonomy of Problem-Based Learning Methods. *Medical Education*, 23: 542–558.

Barrows, H.S. (1988) *The Tutorial Process*. Springfield: Southern Illinois University School of Medicine.

Barrows, H.S. (1996) Problem-Based Learning in Medicine and Beyond: A Brief Overview, in L. Wilkerson and W.H. Gijselaers (eds), *Bringing Problem-Based Learning to Higher Education: Theory and Practice*. San Francisco: Jossey-Bass Inc.

Bayley, L., Bhatnagar, N. and Ellis, P. (2001) Facilitating Information Management Skills and Dispositions, in E. Rideout (ed.), *Transforming Nursing Education through Problem-Based Learning*. Sudbury: Jones and Bartlett Publishers.

Bechtel, G.A., Davidhizer, R. and Bradshaw, M.J. (1999) Problem-Based Learning in a Competency-Based World. *Nurse Education Today*, 19: 182–187.

Beer, S. (1979) *The Heart of the Enterprise*. Chichester: John Wiley and Sons.

Belasco, J.A. (1992) *Teaching the Elephant to Dance: Empowering Change in Your Organization*. London: Century Business.

Biggs, J. (1978) Individual and Group Differences in Study Processes. *British Journal of Educational Psychology*, 48: 266–279.

Biggs, J. (1985) The Role of Metalearning in Study Processes. *British Journal of Educational Psychology*, 55: 185–212.

Bignell, J., Groves, H. and Bayley, L. (2001) Developing Learning and Library Resources, in E. Rideout (ed.), *Transforming Nursing Education through Problem-Based Learning*. Sudbury: Jones and Bartlett Publishers.

Biley, F.C. and Smith, K.L. (1998) 'The Buck Stops Here': Accepting Responsibility for Learning and Actions after Graduation for a Problem-Based Learning Nursing Education Curriculum. *Journal of Advanced Nursing*, 27: 1021–1029.

Blake, J. (1994) Library Resources for Problem-Based Learning: The Programme Perspective. *Computer Methods and Programmes in Biomedicine*, 44: 167–173.

Blumberg, P. and Michael, J.A. (1992) Development of Self-Directed Learning Behaviours in a Partially Teacher-Directed Problem-Based Learning Curriculum. *Teaching and Learning in Medicine*, 4 (1): 3–8.

Brookfield, S.D. (1986) *Understanding and Facilitating Adult Learning*. Milton Keynes: Open University Press.

Brookfield, S.D. (1993) *Developing Critical Thinkers*. Milton Keynes: Open University Press.

Bruce, A. and Langdon, K. (2000) *Project Management*. London: Dorling Kindersley.

Cannon, C.A. and Schell, K.A. (2001) Problem-Based Learning: Preparing Nurses for Practice, in B.J. Duch, S.E. Groh and D.E. Allen (eds), *The Power of Problem-Based Learning*. Virginia: Stylus Publishing.

Chase, R.L. (1991) The 70% Solution. *The TQM Magazine*, 3 (2): 67.

Clark, S. (2001) Student Learning Styles in the Mediated Environment: WebCT and the Adult Learner, in the Third Annual WebCT Conference: Transforming the Educational Experience. Vancouver, B.C., Canada: June 23–27, 2001.

Cleverly, D. (1995) A Critical Investigation into the Relationship Between How Students on the BSc (Hons) Nursing Degree Course 'Learn How to Learn' and the Way that Metalearning is Influenced by Educators, unpublished thesis, University of Greenwich.

Cole, G.A. (1996) *Management: Theory and Practice*. London: Letts Educational.

Coles, C. (1998) Is Problem-Based Learning the Only Way? in D. Boud and G. Feletti (eds), *The Challenge of Problem-Based Learning*. London: Kogan Page.

Communication and Information Technology Services (2001) *An Introduction to WebCT*. Chelmsford: APU.

Cooke, M. (1995) Integrating Knowledge in Clinical Practice, in C. Alavi (ed.), *Problem-Based Learning in a Health Sciences Curriculum*. London: Routledge.

Creedy, D. and Hand, B. (1994) The Implementation of Problem-Based Learning: Changing Pedagogy in Nurse Education. *Journal of Advanced Nursing*, 20: 696–702.

Creedy, D., Horsfall, J. and Hand, B. (1992) Problem-Based Learning in Nurse Education: An Australian View. *Journal of Advanced Nursing*, 17: 727–733.

Crosby, P.B. (1979) *Quality is Free*. New York: McGraw-Hill Book Company.

David, T., Patel, L. and Burdett, K. (1999) *Problem-Based Learning in Medicine*. London: Royal Society of Medicine Press Ltd.

Davies, P. (1991) What Does the Future Hold? *TQM Magazine*, 3 (3): 141–143.

Davis, W.K., Nairn, R., Paine, M.E., Anderson, R.M. and Oh, M.S. (1992) Effects of Expert and Non-Expert Facilitators on the Small Group Process and on Student Performance. *Academic Medicine*, 67 (7): 470–474.

Day, C., Fraser, D., Mallik, M., Astor, L., Cooper, M., Hall, C., Hallawell, B. and Narayanasamy, A. (1998) *Research Highlights: The Role of the Teacher/Lecturer in Practice*. London: ENB.

De Graaff, E. (1993) Introduction: The Principles of Problem-Based Learning, in E. de Graaff and P.A.J. Bouhuijs (eds), *Implementation of Problem-Based Learning in Higher Education*. Amsterdam: Thesis Publishers.

De Grave, W.S., Dolmans, D.H.J.M. and Van der Vleuten, C.P.M. (1999) Profiles of the Effective Tutors in Problem-Based Learning: Scaffolding Student Learning. *Medical Education*, 33: 901–906.

Dearing, R. (1997) Higher Education in the Learning Society. The National Committee of Inquiry into Higher Education for Nursing. Online. Available HTTP: <http://www.leeds. ac.uk/educol/ncihe/docsinde.htm> (accessed 14 August 2002).

Department of Health (1989) *A Strategy for Nursing*. London: Department of Health Nursing Division.

Department of Health (1999) *Making a Difference – Strengthening the Nursing, Midwifery and Health Visiting Contribution to Health and Healthcare*. London: DH.

Dolmans, D.H.J.M., Wolfhagen, A.P. and Van der Vleuten, C. (2001) Why Aren't They Working? in P. Schwartz, S. Mennin and G. Webb (eds), *Problem-Based Learning Case Studies, Experience and Practice*. London: Kogan Page.

Doring, A., Bramwell-Vial, A. and Bingham, B. (1995) Staff Comfort/Discomfort with Problem-Based Learning: A Preliminary Study. *Nurse Education Today*, 15: 263–266.

Duch, B.J. and Groh, S.E. (2001) *Assessment Strategies in a Problem-Based Learning Course*. Virginia: Stylus Publishing.

Ebersole, S. (1995) Media Determinism in Cyberspace. Online. Available HTTP: <http://www.regent.edu/acad/schcom/rojc/mdic/mcluhan.html> (accessed 19 August 2002).

Engle, C.E. (1998) Not Just a Method But a Way of Life, in D. Boud and G. Feletti (eds), *The Challenge of Problem-Based Learning*. London: Kogan Page.

English National Board for Nursing, Midwifery and Health Visiting (1994) *Creating Lifelong Learners. Partnerships for Care: Guidelines for Pre-Registration Nursing Programmes of Education*. London: ENB.

English National Board for Nursing, Midwifery and Health Visiting (2000) *Education in Focus: Strengthening Pre-Registration Nursing and Midwifery Education*. London: ENB.

Feletti, G. (1993) Inquiry-Based and Problem-Based Learning: How Similar are these Approaches to Nursing and Medical Education? *Higher Education Research and Development*, 12 (2): 143–156.

Fogarty, R. (1997) *Problem-Based Learning and Other Curriculum Models for the Multiple Intelligences Classroom*. Illinois: Sky Light Training and Publishing Inc.

Friere, P. (1972) *Pedagogy of the Oppressed*. Middlesex: Penguin Education.

Frost, M. (1996) An Analysis of the Scope and Value of Problem-Based Learning in the Education of Health Care Professionals. *Journal of Advanced Nursing*, 24: 1047–1053.

Garrigan, P. (1997) Facilitating Effective Student-Centred Learning: Enablement and Ennoblement. *Journal of Further and Higher Education*, 21 (1): 97–105.

Gibbon, C. (1998) Problem-Based Learning: Giving Control to the Student. *Nursing Times Learning Curve*, 2 (4): 4–5.

Gijselaers, W.H. (1996) Connecting Problem-Based Practices with Educational Theory, in L. Wilkerson and W.H. Gijselaers (eds), *Bringing Problem-Based Learning to Higher Education: Theory and Practice*. San Francisco: Jossey-Bass Inc.

Glasgow, N.A. (1997) *New Curriculum for New Times: A Guide to Student-Centred, Problem-Based Learning*. London: Sage Publications Ltd.

Gordon, J.R., Mondy, R.W., Sharplin, A. and Premeaux, S.R. (1990) *Management and Organizational Behaviour*. Boston: Allyn and Bacon.

Gross, R.D. (1990) *Psychology: The Science of Mind and Behaviour*. London: Hodder and Stoughton.

Habermas, J. (1978) *Knowledge and Human Interests*. London: Heinemann Educational Books Ltd.

Haith-Cooper, M. (2000) Problem-Based Learning within Health Professional Education: What is the Role of the Lecturer? A Review of the Literature. *Nurse Education Today*, 20: 267–272.

Harris, C. (1996) Academic Support Service, in D. Warner and D. Palfreyman (eds), *Higher Education Management: The Key Elements*. Buckingham: Open University Press.

Hart, M. (1985) Thematization of Power, the Search for Common Interests, and Self-Reflection: Towards a Comprehensive Concept of Emancipatory Education. *International Journal of Lifelong Education*, 4 (2): 119–134.

Hendry, G.D., Frommer, M. and Walker, R.A. (1999) Constructivism and Problem-Based Learning. *Journal of Further and Higher Education*, 23 (3): 359–371.

Hitchcock, M.A., Stritter, F.T. and Bland, C.J. (1993) Faculty Development in the Health Professions: Conclusions and Recommendations. *Medical Teacher*, 14 (4): 295–309.

Integrated Technologies, Inc. (2002) Cone of Learning (Edgar Dale). Online. Available HTTP: <http://www.intech.com/education/training.htm> (accessed 23 July 2002).

Jackson, M. and Parker, S. (1998) The Role of Library and Information Services in Supporting Students in Research-Based Learning: Some Findings of the IMPEL2 Project. *Journal of Further and Higher Education*, 22 (2): 173–181.

Jones, J.A. (1985) A Study of Nurse Tutors' Conceptualization of their Ward Teaching Role. *Journal of Advanced Nursing*, 10: 349–360.

Jowett, S. (1995) Added Value. *Nursing Times*, 91 (1): 55–57.

Knowles, M. (1983) Andragogy: An Emerging Technology for Adult Learning, in M. Tight (ed.), *Adult Learning and Education*. Beckenham: Croom-Helm Ltd.

Knowles, M.C. (1990) *The Adult Learner: A Neglected Species*. Houston: Gulf Publishing Company.

Koltay, Z. and Calhoun, K. (2002) Designing For WOW!: The Optimal Information Gateway. Online. Available HTTP: <http://www.ala.org/acrl/koltay.pdf> (accessed 27 July 2002).

Lathlean, J. (1987) Are You Prepared to be a Staff Nurse? *Nursing Times*, 83 (36): 25–27.

Lawton, D. (1981) Curriculum Evaluation, in P. Gordon (ed.), *The Study of the Curriculum*. London: Batsford Academic and Educational Ltd.

Little, S. (1998) Preparing Tertiary Teachers for Problem-Based Learning, in D. Boud and G. Feletti (eds), *The Challenge of Problem-Based Learning*. London: Kogan Page.

Long, G., Grandis, S. and Glasper, E.A. (1999) Investing in Practice: Enquiry and Problem-Based Learning. *British Journal of Nursing*, 8(17): 1171–1174.

Luker, K., Carlisle, C. and Kirk, S. (1995) *Research Highlights: The Evolving Role of the Nurse Teacher in the Light of Educational Reform*. London: ENB.

Magnussen, L., Ishida, D. and Itano, J. (2000) The Impact of the Use of Inquiry-Based Learning as a Teaching Methodology of the Development of Critical Thinking. *Journal of Nursing Education*, 39 (8): 360–364.

Maitland, B. and Cowdray, R. (2001) Redesigning PBL: Resolving the Integration Problem, in P. Schwartz, S. Mennin and G. Webb (eds), *Problem-Based Learning Case Studies, Experience and Practice.* London: Kogan Page.

Marshall, J.G., Fitzgerald, D., Busby, L. and Heaton, G. (1993) A Study of Library Use in Problem-Based and Traditional Medical Curricula. *Bulletin of the Medical Library Association*, 81 (3): 299–305.

Martin, E. and Ramsden, P. (1987) Learning Skills or Skill in Learning, in J. Richardson, M. Eysenck and D. Piper (eds), *Student Learning.* Milton Keynes: Open University Press.

Marton, F. and Säljö, R. (1976) On Qualitative Differences in Learning: 11 – Outcome as a Function of the Learner's Conception of the Task. *British Journal of Educational Psychology*, 4 (6): 4–11.

Mezirow, J. (1983) A Critical Theory of Adult Learning and Education, in M. Tight (ed.), *Adult Learning and Education.* Beckenham: Croom Helm Ltd.

Mezirow, J. (1991) *Transformative Dimensions of Adult Learning.* Oxford: Jossey-Bass Publishers.

Miller, D. (1990) *The Icarus Paradox: How Exceptional Companies Bring About their Own Downfall.* New York: Harper Business Publisher.

Milligan, F. (1999) Beyond the Rhetoric of Problem-Based Learning: Emancipatory Limits and Links with Androgogy. *Nurse Education Today*, 19: 548–555.

Murray, I. and Savin-Baden, M. (2000) Staff Development in Problem-Based Learning. *Teaching in Higher Education*, 5 (1): 107–126.

National Health Service Executive (1998) *1. Changes in Pre-Registration Nursing and Midwifery Degree Commissions. 2. Extension of Practice Placements to All Pre-Registration Nursing and Midwifery Students.* Health Service Circular. 2 September 1998.

Nayer, M. (1995) Faculty Development for Problem-Based Learning Programmes. *Teaching and Learning in Medicine*, 7 (3): 138–148.

Peters, M. (2000) Does Constructivist Epistemology Have a Place in Nurse Education? *Journal of Nursing Education*, 39 (4): 166–172.

Phillips, L.D. and Phillips, M.C. (1993) Facilitated Work Groups: Theory and Practice. *Journal of the Operational Research Society*, 44 (6): 533–549.

Ramsden, P. and Entwistle, N.J. (1981) Effects of Academic Departments on Students' Approaches to Studying. *British Journal of Educational Psychology*, 51: 368–383.

Rankin, J. (1992) Problem-Based Medical Education: Effect on Library Use? *Bulletin of the Medical Library Association*, 80: 36–43.

Rankin, J.A. (1996) Problem-Based Learning and Libraries: A Survey of the Literature. *Health Libraries Review*, 13: 33–42.

Rideout, E. and Carpio, B. (2001) The Problem-Based Learning Model of Nursing Education, in E. Rideout (ed.), *Transforming Nursing Education through Problem-Based Learning.* London: Jones and Bartlett Publishing International.

Rogers, C. (1983) *Freedom to Learn for the 80's.* Columbus: Charles E. Merrill Publishing Company.

Rogers, C.R. (1980) *A Way of Being.* Boston: Houghton Mifflin Company.

Rogers, P. (1995) Self-Assessment of Project 2000 Supervision. *Nursing Times*, 91 (39): 42–45.

Ross, B. (1995) What Lessons – and Where To? in C. Alavi (ed.), *Problem-Based Learning in a Health Sciences Curriculum.* London: Routledge.

Royle, J.A., Sword, W., Black, M., Brown, B. and Carr, T. (2001) Developing Clinical Opportunities and Resources for Problem-Based Learning, in E. Rideout (ed.), *Transforming Nursing Education through Problem-Based Learning*. London: Jones and Bartlett Publishers International.

Ryan, G. (1998) Ensuring the Students Develop an Adequate, and Well-Structured, Knowledge Base, in D. Boud and G. Feletti (eds), *The Challenge of Problem-Based Learning*. London: Kogan Page.

Salvin, R.E. (1996) Research on Cooperative Learning and Achievement: What We Know, What We Need to Know. *Contemporary Educational Psychology*, 21: 43–69.

Savery, J.R. and Duffy, T.M. (1995) Problem-Based Learning: An Instructional Model and its Constructivist Framework. *Educational Technology*, 35: 31–38.

Schein, E.H. (2001) Kurt Lewin's Change Theory in the Field and in the Classroom: Notes Towards a Model of Managed Learning. Online. Available HTTP: <http://www.a2zpsychology.com/articles/kurt_lewin's_change_theory.htm> (accessed 29 July 2002).

Schwartz, P., Mennin, S. and Webb, G. (2001) *Problem-Based Learning: Case Studies, Experience and Practice*. London: Kogan Page.

Shah, I. (1990) *The Way of the Sufi*. London: Penguin Group.

Shand, M. (1987) The Staff Nurse: Unreasonable Expectations? *Nursing Times*, 83 (36): 28–80.

Smith, R. (1983) *Learning How to Learn*. Milton Keynes: The Open University Press.

Sweeney, J.F.C. (1986) Nurse Education: Learner-Centred or Teacher-Centred? *Nurse Education Today*, 6: 257–262.

The Learn Website Authors (1998) NCSU's Undergraduate Learning Handbook. Online. Available HTTP: <http://www.ncsu.edu/learn/saying.html> (accessed 21 June 2002).

Thomsett, M.C. (2002) *The Little Black Book of Project Management*. New York: AMACOM.

United Kingdom Central Council (1986) *Project 2000: A New Preparation for Practice*. London: UKCC.

United Kingdom Central Council (1999) *Fitness for Practice*. London: UKCC.

University Health Sciences Librarians (2001) 'Making a Difference': Contributions of Higher Education Library and Information Professionals to the Government's Nursing, Midwifery and Health Visiting Strategy. Online. Available HTTP: <http://www.uhsl.ac.uk/reports/mad.html> (accessed 19 August 2002).

Van Niekerk, K. and Van Aswegen, E. (1993) Implementing Problem-Based Learning in Nursing. *Nursing RSA Verpleging*, 8 (5): 37–41.

Wakeham, M. (2000) The Library and Inquiry-Based Learning. *North Circular*, Newsletter of the Library and Information Development Unit, 27: 10–12. Anglia Polytechnic University.

Walton, H.J. and Matthews, M.B. (1989) Essentials of Problem-Based Learning. *Medical Education*, 23: 542–558.

WebCT (2002) Online Learning for the Entire Enterprise. Online. Available HTTP: <http://www.webct.com/products/viewpage?name=products_campus_edition> (accessed 19 August 2002).

White, E., Davies, S., Twinn, S. and Riley, E. (1993) *Research Highlights: A Detailed Study of the Relationships between Teaching, Support, Supervision and Role Modelling for Students in Clinical Areas within the Context of Project 2000 Course*. London: ENB.

Wilkerson, L. (1996) Tutors and Small Groups in Problem-Based Learning: Lessons from the Literature, in L. Wilkerson and W.H. Gijselaers (eds), *Bringing Problem-Based Learning to Higher Education: Theory and Practice.* San Francisco: Jossey-Bass Inc.

Wilkerson, L. and Hundert, E.M. (1998) Becoming a Problem-Based Tutor: Increasing Self-Awareness Through Faculty Development, in D. Boud and G. Feletti (eds), *The Challenge of Problem-Based Learning.* London: Kogan Page.

Wilkie, K. (2000) The Nature of Problem-Based Learning, in S. Glen and K. Wilkie (eds), *Problem-Based Learning in Nursing.* London: Macmillan Press Ltd.

Willis, J. (1996) The Placement Dilemma. *Nursing Times,* 92 (5): 55–58.

Woods, D. R. (1994) *Problem-Based Learning: How to Gain the Most from PBL.* Ontario: Donald R. Woods.

World Health Organization (1993) *Increasing the Relevance of Education for Health Professionals.* Geneva: WHO Technical Report Series 838.

Zeitz, H.J. and Paul, H. (1993) Facilitator Expertise and Problem-Based Learning in PBL and Traditional Curricula. *Academic Medicine,* 68 (3): 203–204.

Index